What others are saying . . .

"Like most with a very busy schedule and challenging work demands, I do not have a lot of time to shop for 'the perfect outfit,' which often leads to stress, especially since a major aspect of my job is attending public functions. If you are like me and have ever said 'I hate my body in these clothes!' then Wendy Lyn's book is a must read. *Naked to Knockout* is a book every woman needs on her nightstand, her dresser, and near her closet!"

—**KENDRA AKERS,** *President of Akers Media Group and Publisher of* Style *and* Healthy Living *Magazines*

"Beautifully written and from the heart. From the first page you can hear Wendy teaching, guiding, and showing you the how and why of looking great and being your best. Filled with examples and stories, you'll learn how to make yourself look your best and achieve that victory!"

—**ANN MCINDOO,** *Author,* So, You Want to Write!

"I've been a working professional in theatre for over 40 years and have seen many facets of the self-image issues that women face today. Our society seems to only look at the surface, especially in the entertainment industry, where false or fleeting adulation can cause a woman to lose sight of who she really is. Wendy's way of helping women balance the interior and the exterior is very accessible. Readers will not only be enlightened but also entertained and will come to love this delightful woman that I have been fortunate enough to call my friend for a majority of my life."

—**CHRISTOPHER AYRES,** *Actor/Director, Houston, Texas*

"Everybody needs to understand the impact of this silent deal-killer. Image matters, and Wendy Lyn is the perfect person to make sure that your image says 'deal maker,' not 'deal breaker'! Her book will help you step up your image and improve overall. She knows her stuff and intuitively knows how to teach it."

—**ALLAN BORESS,** *CPA; Author,* The "I Hate Selling" Book; *National Speaker; and Consultant*

"If you want to save time and money while owning a knockout wardrobe, this is the book for you. I highly recommend Wendy Lyn's approach to blending your inner and outer beauty, from clothes, to hair, makeup, and accessories. She unlocks the mystery of style and shows that you don't have to spend a fortune to look terrific. And when you're done reading it, you'll have a 'wow' style all your own."

—**KATHLEEN HAWKINS,** *Founder and President, WOAMTEC*

"From the moment I met Wendy Lyn, I could tell that she was someone I wanted in my professional circle. Her personal presence is polished, and her warmth and sincerity is evident. More time with her has simply confirmed my initial impressions. Combined with her professional knowledge, her energy and love for her work is contagious. We could all use a little N2K help".

—**JULIE BAUKE,** *Author of* Stop Peeing On Your Shoes, *Coach & CEO, Congruity Career Consulting, Cincinnati*

"Wendy Lyn is a dynamic communicator! If you want someone who knows how to engage any audience by using appropriate humor, material that connects, and does so in a motivating style all her own, I recommend you experience her passion for people today. Her intuitive leadership and life experience makes her message life changing for many!"

—**DR. HAL KITCHINGS,** *Pastor and Teacher*

NAKED TO KNOCKOUT

NAKED TO KNOCKOUT

Beauty from the Inside Out

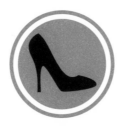

Embrace your unique image, style,

and fashion sense

WENDY LYN PHILLIPS

WENDY LYN INC.
EUSTIS, FL

Published by
Wendy Lyn Inc.
Eustis, FL
www.NakedtoKnockout.com

Publisher's Cataloging-in-Publication Data
Phillips, Wendy Lyn.

    Naked to knockout beauty from the inside out : embrace your unique image, style, and fashion sense / Wendy Lyn Phillips.—Eustis, FL : Wendy Lyn Inc., 2012.

    p. ; cm.

    ISBN13: 978-0-9852725-0-0

    1. Beauty, Personal. 2. Fashion. 3. Clothing and dress. 4. Cosmetics. I. Title.

    GT499.P55 2012
    646.72—dc22   2011961336

FIRST EDITION

Project coordination by Jenkins Group, Inc.
www.BookPublishing.com

Cover and Interior design by Chris Rhoads
Full Color Insert design by Brooke Camfield
Interior layout by Brooke Camfield

Printed in the United States of America
16   15   14   13   12 • 5   4   3   2   1

Dedication

This book is dedicated to my family. To my parents who have loved me unconditionally and made sacrifices so that my life could be beautiful. To Mackenzie and Kendall . . . I imagined you long before I knew you, and your reality is God's most beautiful gift to me. To Glenn, thank you for being the wind beneath my wings and stepping up to be the best father our girls could have. Your love for me inside and out is really what made this book possible.

Contents

OBSTACLE OR OPPORTUNITY?

Do you like what you see when you look in the mirror?

I realize some days may be better than others, but we all have at least a few good hair days, right? How we deal with the bad hair days has taught me a lesson about life, a lesson I like to refer to as the "Obstacle or Opportunity Option," which is really about what perspective I choose to have about "this" situation, this job, this reflection I see in the mirror. I have the option of looking in the mirror and seeing obstacles that hinder me, or I have the option of seeing opportunities that strengthen me. The options are always there, but I've had to learn to strip away all the cover-ups and move the obstacles out of the way so that I can get down to the naked truth and see the positive possibilities.

Don't we all?

Liking what you see in the mirror goes far deeper and is more valuable than what's visible at first glance. There's much more to your appearance than a single glance because there's much more to YOU than that. And how we *value* something (or someone) affects how we see it. Ultimately, how we value what we see in the mirror affects how others see us. The value you give yourself is the value others will generally assign to you. A confident woman has a special way of making those around her feel better about themselves, too. Don't believe me? What happens to the mood in a room when a real grouch walks in? Everyone's mood sinks. The opposite is true as well; when a confident woman walks in, her character and integrity lift others' moods, and in their eyes, her likeability meter ticks up a little higher. When that happens, more people find her attractive.

There's no doubt that a person with character and integrity is attractive to those who know him or her well. But what distinguishes those we think are beautiful based on a first impression from those who become more beautiful to us over time? We have to define it first.

The definition of true beauty is so controversial that it's easier to simply say that it's "in the eye of the beholder." When I surveyed one hundred women on their definition of what a truly beautiful woman was, the only actual person they named was either their own mother or a close family member. One hundred percent of them connected character traits to their definition of true beauty. We're not talking about the head-turning, mouth-dropping works of art. Although we've all seen those types and can name at least a handful, I'm talking about the everyday woman with no touch-ups or airbrushed head shots: the working moms who sacrifice sleep to get up before work and go to the gym, the stay-home moms who are up all night with a wee one who's afraid of the thunder or has an earache, and the women who forfeit careers later in life to take care of their own aging parents in lieu of putting them in a facility. These women are doing worthy things that are aligned with pure beauty. There are millions of you out there, all with your own beautiful story to tell. You're not being asked to tell your story on the *Good Morning America, The View or Oprah's OWN network* because it's just not perceived as that juicy or entertaining.

While you might not be on camera, though, you are on stage every day playing the role of CEO, taxi cab driver, nurse, and VIP in someone's life. Someone would simply cry or die if you weren't in the car line to pick up him or her at school. Someone would have a total come apart if you didn't know the right blankie to send to the nursery. Someone would miss your reassuring smile from the bleachers if you weren't there. Someone would frown all week if you missed the visits and calls that he or she has become so accustomed to. Yes, these are the "Everyday Housewives," not the "Desperate" ones; the only thing you're desperate for is a little recognition, appreciation, and passionate love. And how deserving you are! This book will affirm your position whether you're single, a stay-home mom, a business executive, an empty nester, or a silver fox. It will help you go from naked to knockout on a daily basis and do it from the inside out! The value we give ourselves is the message we send out, and it all starts with what's inside.

Getting your outer shell and image to reflect your inner beauty is something most women find challenging. Merging the two is the ultimate goal, and that's just where I come in. Whether your focus is to grow your business or to grow your community and family, you really can't empower others unless YOU LOOK empowering. And when you look good, you feel good. Having something to give means you must first be filled up with substance on the inside. After all, tipping a teapot that's empty means you're going to be disappointed if you're expecting a fabulous afternoon high tea experience.

This void, this obsession with what's on the outside while airbrushing away what's on the inside, is a big reason I chose to write on this topic. I've seen enough lies passed on from a knockout "teapot" who had nothing more than superficial hot air to contribute to any conversation. And I myself have bought the lies that promised popularity, success, and peace. A beautiful woman who focuses on outer beauty alone and who does not love herself is limited in her ability to love others, including our creator. God created us all to love fully, to experience abundance, and to do it with a muscle that is often developed through trials. You simply cannot have beauty on the outside alone, with a dark, cold, and ugly inside. No one admires that.

What others admire is someone who possesses qualities such as honesty, service, compassion, balance, confidence, strength, charisma, warmth, and grace. It's been said that a true beauty is one without any makeup or clothes on. Well, even that is controversial! It is my belief that as your outer style reflects an inner core based on the qualities mentioned above, you become naturally beautiful regardless of aesthetics. This chasm between the two is where I will build some bridges for every woman to walk across with increased confidence. Are you ready to connect your inner beauty to your outer image and BE that woman whom others admire?

I can help you improve your self-confidence by blending your inner beauty and your outer beauty so that you'll experience these three benefits:

1. You will have deeper and more meaningful relationships because allowing others to get to know the real you will be a treasure. *No more masking who you are so you can try to appear like someone you aren't.*

2. You will save time and money getting dressed every day because you'll learn what works for you and stop buying what doesn't. *Creating a style all your own includes providing the optimum in "dressing for success" options: flattering to your figure, colors that enhance, and accessories to add pizzazz.*

3. You will have a classic makeup look so you can dash out the door in minutes. *Your makeup will achieve a quick and classy style, and you'll wear what's in your cases and drawers because you'll have the appropriate products and colors to enhance. Knowing your own style and reflecting it will become easy.*

No, your brand is not your logo, your business card, or what's on your Web site. YOU are your brand, and you are selling YOU long before you are selling a product or service. Your overall image either draws others to you or drives them away. It opens up doors in networking, at the store, and at the salon, with the principal, your boss, or the mail carrier. These are examples of relationships that may be strengthened with an improved image and style. And what if receiving superb customer service versus average service actually depended on you? The message you send with your appearance is speaking loud and clear long before you utter any words. Why does this matter so much?

Is there anyone you know who wouldn't agree that what's on the inside matters more than what's on the outside? And yet, after twenty-some years in the beauty industry, I've got an ugly, naked truth to share with you whether you want to hear it or not: people aren't often drawn to you enough to experience the blessing of what you have to offer if they are not FIRST drawn to your external style.

Finding a way to fluidly balance these two criteria is not an easy task. We can give an exuberant amount of attention to the internal and neglect the external and vice versa. As a young girl, I found it very appealing to overindulge in my outer shell. Even when I knew better, it was always easier to give in to feelings of inadequacy over principles of value. Having designer clothes poses no definitive change to who you really are, but the gratifying feeling of importance that comes as a result of wearing them can be confusing. Being driven by feelings alone can get ugly. Some women I know rack up credit card debts from spending unnecessarily to satisfy their drive to have the latest, hottest, just-released whatever: designer purse, jeans, jewelry, or shoes. Their appetite for more takes over. I guess that's normal; what isn't normal is continuing that extreme behavior with detrimental results. That's insane. And you've heard the definition of that, right?

***Insanity = doing the same thing over and over
but expecting different results.***

Have you ever been there? Of course you have. We all have circumstances and issues to overcome, and looking back into our past helps bring some clarity to the way we have been affected. Some children with difficult pasts of abuse, divorce, disorders, abandonment, neglect, and the like rise above all odds to accomplish more than others with simpler backgrounds, and yet others with that same troubled past can stay defeated in the cycle and continue to pass on an unhealthy legacy.

The chain can be broken. Looking at the past for clarity can help, as long as we remember that we have options on how to move forward. Seeing the past as an obstacle to progress results in no action, no change, no improvement. Ah, but if I choose to see the obstacle as an opportunity for change, an opportunity to turn something unwanted into something beneficial, well, then, there's progress. There's *hope*.

Trust me: I speak from experience. The parent-child relationship bears a huge impact on how a child views his or her worth. It takes on many forms . . . and I should know. It was Christmastime; I was twenty years old, enjoying the break from college with my family on vacation in Virginia. That's when I shockingly and accidentally met my biological father for the first time. (Or so I thought; I was stunned to learn that my parents had divorced when I was barely three, and I had no memory of him whatsoever.) This was not MY divine plan, and to say that it took quite a while to adjust to this revelation would certainly be an understatement. The decision to choose an opportunity or an obstacle was solely mine, although I didn't fully "get" it at the time. After months of unsettled sleep and disappointment with what I saw as an intrusion, I obliged him and his wife with a Thanksgiving visit across the state lines.

As I sat in a very crowded airport that day, it seemed that I really was the only one in the whole terminal to hear the loudspeaker: "Wendy Lyn, do you want this to be an opportunity or an obstacle that you bang your head against for the rest of your life?"

I didn't need a two-by-four upside the head to figure out the answer. Being an over-comer isn't easy, but it was the only decision for me. That "AHA" moment defined some future decisions for me that I had no idea were coming. You just don't know when the Mack trucks of bad luck, bad breaks, and heartaches will come, but they all started heading my way. That's what happens with intrusions. They leave the door open just enough for lots of other things to come in, too.

Dealing with a new family dynamic was challenging to say the least. From my selfish view, it certainly seemed unfair that I was the one having to be inconvenienced. Isn't that the way it usually happens? The inconveniences of life happen at the most inopportune times.

During my college years, my goals were quite simple: go to college, expect the message from God to be loud (and include an outline of what I was to do with my life, as long as it agreed with my list), have Mr. Right ride in on a white horse, marry him, start a family, and be a stay-home mom. Well . . . maybe have my own business, too. I always was the entrepreneurial type. Notice the list did not include my biological father entering center stage, or even backstage.

After my AHA moment, I decided to put on my big-girl pants and embrace the kink in my plans. I had to recognize that much of my confidence and security had come from performance-based arenas that I could easily control, such as sports and volunteering and academics (which is why I excelled at them all). This was different. Topsy-turvy. Cattywampus, as they say down South. It was like walking into my room and finding everything had been set on a slight tilt; I was facing downhill and trying not to fall over. I do like the wind in my face, but being suddenly thrown into an arena that I clearly could not control, could not explain easily to others, and was not comfortable in was a bit much. My beliefs, motives, worth, and more were challenged to the hilt by this new involvement, and all of it eventually resulted in being a huge blessing.

Why do I say that?

It goes back to having options and choosing how to view things. I've had lots of other difficult circumstances and uncomfortable situations over the past two decades, and I'll have more in the next two. What I've learned is that I am free to choose to accept the circumstances in my life as opportunities rather than obstacles, no matter how bad they are, so that I can grow through them. I choose to look for ways to improve myself, my circumstances, and my relationships.

And you can, too. It's a choice. As the old saying goes, **you can either be better or be bitter.** This lesson is one I am grateful to have learned. I will pass it on in a powerful way to my daughters and to anyone else whose bitterness is chained to a past he or she cannot control.

And as for me and my "intrusion"? It's been twenty-four years, and I am happy to say that accepting others for decisions they have made is both healing and helpful for all involved. It's been a hoot and a joy getting to know my biological dad and his wife, and they are enjoying their grandchildren immensely. All is not perfect, but what family is? I wouldn't have changed it. And in the process of learning to accept him, I've learned that acceptance of yourself—your faults, sins, mistakes, nakedness, and all—is even more helpful. Forgiveness is a beautiful thing!

"You have two primary choices in life: to accept conditions as they exist, or accept the responsibility for changing them."—Denis Waitley

As I write this, I can see the impact that choosing to embrace the new family relationship has had on my life, and it's ultimately been for the better. I also see how easily I could have chosen not to accept things, and I am convinced that that would have set a pattern for stubbornly focusing on obstacles—I can't or won't accept this and move forward—a pattern that would have led to accepting more and more obstacles "as is" rather than choosing to overcome them.

Too often we opt for the status quo rather than pursuing the potential that lies just beyond. To maintain status quo, we often blame others for the way our life is and don't take responsibility for doing anything about it. When my unexpected Christmas present appeared, my own self-image was at an all-time low due to poor relationship choices I had made and how unfulfilling they'd proved to be. I was desperately searching for the real me. My new family dynamic was the icing on the cake that turned everything I'd ever known to be true upside down. I longed to rewind the bad movie and go back to the scene with my happy, traditional *Leave It to Beaver* family. You know what I'm talking about! The one-mother, one-father, one-younger-sister, one-dog, and no-big-life-decisions-to-make kind of life, but I couldn't. I couldn't control it, I couldn't change it, I couldn't rewind anything.

That was in the eighties, when what I was clinging to was pretty much still the average "normal" family unit. Today, "normal" is so loosely used; what once was deemed "odd" is now the new normal. There are as many family unit variations as there are shades of blue.

I had to let go of what I thought defined my value, namely, my achievements. Awards, approval, appearances, whatever—the perfect world I'd contrived for myself was no longer valid, and I had a choice to make about who I was and what defined me: Perfection? Or something else?

It was an ultimate turning point in my life to accept what I believed to be true since the beginning of time: that God had made me special and one of a kind with certain unique gifts He could use for good. He had allowed this series of events to happen for a reason, and I would trust Him. His living in and through me brought a new reason to care about appearances because I now understood that I represented Him. He knew me and formed me in my mother's womb, formed my body shape and my skinny arms and the flat chest that I hated—all were part of His divine creation. "I indeed knew you and formed you before time began. . . . I knit your tiny fingers together in your mother's womb" (from Psalm 139, paraphrased by me). Among other reasons, the facts that my mother went to the doctor only one time during nine months of pregnancy and that I wasn't deformed or aborted are miracles in and of themselves, and that was enough. God already knew about all of this. And so, on that Thanksgiving Day, in the airport on the way to my "new" family's home, I decided to look for opportunities for good. I began asking myself, "What's good about this? There has to be a way I can use this experience for good." I was beginning to change the way I viewed things. Selah.

The continuing story of how my self-image was shaped to go from naked to knockout, and how you can, too, is what this book is about. Since that day in the airport, the value I chose to give myself didn't produce an instant change, but it has drastically improved over the years. And so has our fantastic, fully blended family. I believe that the unity and respect we all have for each other today are the result of what happens when love prevails. You see, reconciliation is also a beautiful thing. Faced with decisions on every issue from business to family drama, eight years of infertility and multiple miscarriages, deaths, and lots of bad hair days and choosing to like what's in the mirror anyway, I still ask myself that valuable question, "Is this an opportunity for good or an obstacle to confine me?" I bet you guessed the answer: it's an opportunity for good! What I know is that when you approach the disappointments of life with a positive slant, you're ten times more likely to find the good and own it. Believing God is for me, I live by faith, embracing things and even some principles I cannot explain. I just know it works for me and that He is real in my life.

I can't help but think of a great story about two little boys playing in a pile of manure. They were in different rooms but were experiencing the same smell, same texture, same amount . . . You get the scenario? One little boy began to cry bloody murder, kicking and screaming, "Get me outta here!" The other boy started jumping right in the middle of it, throwing manure all over the room. When asked what in the world he was doing, he simply said, "Well, with all this poop, there's gotta be a pony under here somewhere!"

Now that's positive thinking to the max!

How about you? Are you dealing with a pile of poop? Are you willing to dig for a pony?

Take a moment below and write about a specific circumstance in your life that you could benefit by asking yourself the question . . . OOOh, Baby, is this an obstacle or an opportunity?

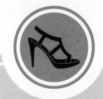

STEP UP TO ACTION:
Find the Pony

My challenging circumstance is

_____

_____

_____

Is this an obstacle or an opportunity?

_____

_____

_____

Are you willing to inspire others? Send me a short story of how you plan to turn obstacles into opportunities and I will send you a free gift!

Go to www.NakedtoKnockout.com and click on Word2Wendy.

Chapter 1

WHY GO FROM GOOD TO GREAT?

Interesting question.

When your "why" is in place, the "how" seems to fall into place a little more easily. I'm not talking about having general contentment in life. I'm talking about stacking the cards in your favor, having an edge on your competition, moving people to action, and standing out in a crowd. So, why go from good to great?

What if I told you that you would get better service 100% of the time when you *look like* you are somebody important? What if I told you that when you stand two equally qualified women next to each other, the one in the skirted suit as opposed to the pants and top will almost always get the job? What if I told you that talking on the phone in business dress as opposed to khakis will make your voice sound more confident, thus resulting in more sales? You may not agree, but studies support all of those claims. Our environment preconditions us to look at appearances alone and make many judgments about a person's level of success. And just what are we judging? For starters, qualities such as trustworthiness, socioeconomic levels and background, educational background, and overall efficiency. Let's face it: it just means you think someone is smarter and can get the job done faster and better when he or she looks the part.

On the road to success in life,
you want to look like you belong there!

Treading water in the pool of mediocrity leads you to accept an average lot in life when life would really have given more. While many are content with just barely getting by and settling for the "good enough" attitude, I have found it so worth the extra effort it takes to be GREAT! Abundance is an option I choose to embrace, and I hope you will, too. It's good to be good . . . but it's better to be great!

> *"The greater danger for most of us lies not in setting our aim too high and falling short, but in setting our aim too low and achieving our mark."*
>
> —Michelangelo

Having a knockout look is easy when you know how and you let it shine through from the inside out. There is a way to avoid making mistakes that could cost you both professionally and socially. Kicking up your image is an investment you make that pays big dividends, and the return on that investment is huge when you learn how to present your best assets to others in a nonmanipulative way, a way that both increases your personal confidence and sends an inviting message.

How we dress is part of our daily visual intake. Appearance says much about you and sends subliminal messages to others long before you have a chance to ever open your mouth. If you're honest, you'll agree that you've formed opinions about others solely based on appearance. It doesn't mean at all that only the most beautiful and attractive get better treatment, but it does mean that if you LOOK like you deserve the best, the best will often come to you. Your attitude, combined with your outward appearance, begets a response that affects your success at anything from a customer service issue to closing a major business deal. Your challenge is to take them both and package them in a way that is attractive to others and uncompromising to your true self.

BEAUTY DEFINED

Mountain sunbeams barely shining through the Bavarian branches laden with snow, a beach sunrise with crashing waves in the background, the birth of your first child, a premium parking spot when you're nine months pregnant, the Prada shoes you've been wanting . . .

on sale, the face and body of Miss America, the perfect cocktail dress, experiencing your child's first competitive win, or simply a good hair day. If you're anything like me, the maturation process has provided more opportunities to find beauty in simple things and yet made it harder to easily define it. According to *Webster's* dictionary, "beauty" can be defined as something that delights the senses or is exciting to the intellect or emotion; something that pleases the mind aesthetically, is of very high standard, and is excellent . . . "This is beautiful."

> *"Though we travel the world over to find the beautiful, we must carry it with us or we find it not."*
>
> —Ralph Waldo Emerson

True beauty is indeed in the eye of the beholder, and it can vary all around the world. In some countries, pale skin and straight blond hair are considered the ultimate standard. Yet, in other countries, dark, bronze, and voluptuous are. It's not just physique that matters. What we all can agree on is that a truly beautiful woman is best defined by a balance of strong inner character that mirrors a strong outer presence; when these two converge, you have beauty in its most organic form . . . consistent at any season of life, in any region of the world. The most beautiful part of the equation is that with this formula, beauty is achievable by all, not just the chosen few who were born with certain traits. **When YOU think of something beautiful, what comes to mind?**

As we unravel this ball of yarn called "beauty," I know that everyone may not agree with my conclusions and positions on some issues. However, that doesn't discredit the journey I have traveled to find them. For some women, all they need to LOOK IN THE MIRROR AND LIKE WHAT THEY SEE is a new "do," a more current wardrobe, or better makeup choices or application tips, and yet other women will like what they see better *simply because they choose to.*

No, we won't be using a microscope to zoom in on every little flaw like so many of us are guilty of doing. Nor are we going to be encouraged to use that concave circus mirror that only makes us look taller and skinnier or shorter and fatter; either way, it lies. We're not going to use any kind of mirror other than a true, honest, reflective one, one that powerful and positive words jump off of. It can actually send encouraging phrases your way. It will tell you that you are worthy, deserving, and capable of so much more than you limit yourself to achieving. This mirror may sound like a fantasy one, but it is one I will continue to sell you throughout the chapters of this book. It is not cheap, and neither are you. Check your price tag. Have you marked yourself down? Get off the clearance rack and get on the display shelves, where your true value can be revealed. You may have to make some very costly trades to own the "I am beautiful and I matter" mirror, but embracing this concept sets the tone for all other principles to follow.

ARE YOU PART OF THE 83%? BE A RENEGADE!

The journey of growing into a beautiful woman is a necessary and normal process from preteen to midlife and even beyond. Without a doubt, it can be a bumpy ride, but a degree of confident beauty is often achieved in direct proportion to the detours we've taken to get there. I don't want to tiptoe through the issues that are obviously challenging women to give in and, worse, give up . . . which can cause huge consequences. When eighty-three percent of women today are unhappy with their body shape and image, it's obvious that confusion about what constitutes "beauty" is running rampant and causing many to chisel, cut, add to, inject, hide, cover up, suck out, pack in, and rearrange body parts all for hope of arriving at what is ultimately proving to be an unhealthy destination.

I say it again: eighty-three percent of women today are unhappy with their body shape and image. That's an outrageous statistic, and we should all be sounding an alarm about the confusing messages we are being fed on the topic of beauty. I hope to change that number by starting with my own family, clientele base, consultants I train, coaching clients, and, ultimately, you, the reader of this book. Being happy with your overall image may be more of a process than a quick decision, but it's also a lot safer and cheaper than chiseling, cutting, adding to, injecting, sucking out, packing in, and rearranging, so hang on and hang in there with me.

VERBAL SELF-ABUSE: CRUSH IT

It's clear we have image issues. The *Today Show* recently reported that most women have thirteen "I hate my body" moments each day. What's up with that? According to Dr. Ann Kearney-Cooke, author of *Change Your Mind, Change Your Body*, whatever you focus on most shapes your brain. We have control over what we think about, and we can choose to say, "Stop!" ***Obsessing about body parts does NOT yield results. Taking action does***. And before you take action, you have to have balanced thinking. Tackling the mental aura is another book altogether, and I will leave it to the folks with all the credentials. My recommendation is that you refer to some really great authors on the subject such as Karl Kuehl, James Dobson, Steve Siebold, Ravi Zacharias, Tony Dungy, Tullian Tchividjian, and Bethany Hamilton.

Bethany teaches us all that body image is strongly connected to what you *choose* to see in the mirror, that "normal" is waaay overrated, and that knowing your purpose in life propels you to succeed regardless of obstacles. Bethany was born to surf. Even though a shark bit off her arm, she was determined to be a national surfing champion . . . and she did it, with sheer determination, a lot of prayer, a lot of soul, and only one arm! She chose not to obsess about a body part. It's a perfect example of reflecting true beauty on the inside and out due in part to the challenges she faced and the life perspective she received through it all.

Creating goals of where you want to go must include things you are passionate about to help offset the depressive serotonin that is released when you walk in drudgery. Allowing the body to release the feel-good hormones called endorphins is an absolute gift you give yourself. They have a dramatic effect on your thought process, enabling you to think more clearly, more realistically, and with purpose—in essence, helping you to clear out the junk in your mind so you can move toward a balanced view of yourself. The other option is to let our feelings guide our actions, and when we do that, we may never get out of bed some days. This will most certainly lead to depression and a faulty self-perception.

Dr. Peter Marzek, a plastic surgeon in central Florida, says that in his practice it is vital that the patient have a realistic expectation of what the intended surgery is going to achieve. "About ninety percent of our clients end up being really good potential patients for cosmetic surgery once the initial consultation is complete," he says. "But when a sixty-something woman brings in her wedding picture and says she wants to look twenty-five again, just like in the picture, I know we have some work to do on the reality of what can be delivered."

The other extreme is also a problem. Dr. Marzek goes on to explain, "The woman that is too critical of herself and sees every little line, flaw, or imperfection is also a bad candidate for surgery. If she lacks that much confidence, surgery isn't going to change anything. You must have a healthy self-image first and see surgery as a simple enhancement to bring out the best you."

If you don't believe me, then believe this esteemed plastic surgeon. If your self-image isn't healthy from the beginning, nothing you do on the outside is going to have a lasting effect. You must learn to be your own best cheerleader. Living with continual verbal abuse from others, and especially from ourselves, sets us up for failure. Self-talk happens almost 24-7, so choose your words wisely. Falling victim to the messages in your head that just are not true is a defeated way to live. I believe one of the biggest reasons women evidently have so many of these unhealthy daily thoughts is that we are so busy serving others that we serve ourselves last with leftovers.

When I am talking to myself and it's headed in a downward spiral, I have learned to ask myself, "Is this really about my body? Is this really even about me? What can I do about this today? Is there a lesson or even a gift here I need or might be missing?" And guess what? Now we're back to the obstacle or opportunity equation again. Those questions usually jar me into another mode of self-talk that causes me to take some action, and ***action always cancels out fear***.

EMPHASIZE YOUR STRENGTHS!

That is, emphasize your own strengths, not someone else's. Women are notorious for comparing their weaknesses to others' strengths. When you do this, you'll always come up short and feeling defeated. It just isn't healthy. If you wished your legs were longer, your hair was straighter, your nose smaller, or your skin clearer, you mustn't focus on those areas. Learn to focus on the one or two other areas that are quite good.

Years ago, before I was married, I began the habit of making a pro-and-con list. It was mostly to help me with business decisions, but eventually I realized that this was a healthy approach to almost any decision. **What we think about we usually bring about**. And whatever gets most of our attention continues to attract more of the same. So you see, YOU'VE GOT SO MUCH MORE POWER TO LOOK IN THE MIRROR AND LIKE WHAT YOU SEE than you actually think! What the mirror reflects is dependent upon what the viewer's ear CHOOSES to hear! Granted, it's never easy when dealing with some of life's most severe struggles, due to accidents, diseases, deformities, and such, and it's from those who have overcome their body shape struggles that we all should find our inspiration. A zit on the end of your nose isn't quite the same as staring at only one arm. Regardless of what you see staring back in your mirror, taking personal responsibility for what you do with it is a great place to start your journey.

By the end of traveling through these pages together, my goal is that you can flat out say: "MIRROR, MIRROR ON THE WALL, WHO'S THE FAIREST OF THEM ALL? GOLLY GEE, IT MUST BE ME, 'CAUSE I'M THE ONLY ONE I SEE!"

Creating a healthy balance of humility and confidence can be a tricky task, and we'll talk more about that in other chapters. For now, *assume an attitude of positive expectancy and begin to embrace the idea that it is worthwhile and possible to possess both.*

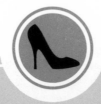

STEP UP TO ACTION:

Self-Quiz

Emphasize your strengths. List at least five qualities you have that are skill-set based and five that are heart qualities:

What I do well (outer character traits)

_____

_____

_____

_____

_____

My heart-quality strengths (inner character—who I am)

_____

_____

_____

_____

_____

_____

1. For your next big decision, make a pro-and-con list. Draw a line down the middle of a piece of paper; on one side, list all the good things about it, and on the other side, list what's not so good and your concerns. Seeing which side stacks up the most supporting statements may help you make the best decision and help you separate feelings from facts.

2. Measure your attitude. Is there a balance of humility and confidence? Which one do you need to exhibit more of?

3. What one realistic step can you take today to improve your body shape? (It can't be to lose 50 pounds! It could be to do 50 sit-ups and 50 squats or walk for 15 minutes, make an appointment with a hairstylist for a new style, buy a new lipstick color, or select a personal coach to hold you accountable.)

The beauty of a woman is not in the clothes she wears, the figure that she carries, or the way she combs her hair.

The beauty of a woman must be seen within her eyes, because that is the doorway to her heart, the place where love resides. The beauty of a woman is not in a facial mole. But true beauty in a woman is reflected in her soul.

It is the caring that she lovingly gives, the passion that she shows, and the beauty of a woman with passing years only grows!

—Audrey Hepburn

Chapter 2

SEXY IN YOUR OWN SKIN

"I hope you have lost your good looks, for while they last any fool can adore you, and the adoration of fools is bad for the soul. No, give me a ruined complexion and a lost figure and sixteen chins on a farmyard of Crow's feet and an obvious wig. Then you shall see me coming out strong." (*attributed to a letter from George Bernard Shaw to Mrs. Patrick Campbell*)

Really? How about that for a love letter! I'm serious. Stop and think . . . could this be true love, directed at a woman's CONTENTS as opposed to her CONTAINER? It's not about what's on the outside, which is fleeting and easily attracts things or people that aren't always in your best interest. He's aware of her beauty but is drawn to her character, a type of character that expresses confidence regardless of how our body changes with age.

How about you? Are you so focused on your *container* that you've forgotten to love your *contents*?

As you read this book, I want you to really think about this: by letting others decide what's truly beautiful (or not) based on your outward looks, you are giving them power—power to influence your thoughts, limit your options, and dismiss your true identity. My heart's desire is that you will choose to keep that power for yourself, because when you do, you really will look in the mirror and like what you see.

Learning to be sexy in your own skin is not about your "container" or skin; it's not about your container's shape, size, color, texture, or anything else. It's about the contents: your personality and especially your character. And for the record, the contents will grow and change and renew and slough off useless layers much the way our skin does, figuratively speaking, of course! There are two sides to this aging process, you know . . . While the outside seems to deteriorate over time, the inside will blossom continually, if you will choose to nurture it. That little bit of wisdom came to me when I reached that big four-oh, thank you very much. As I work with women in their second half of life, I see it all the time: an inner glow from the woman who cares for her husband with a debilitating disease or who has found joy in pursuing a long-deferred goal. The nurturing for your inner glow may need a little fertilizer called self-respect.

Something magical happened at forty. I suddenly became much less interested in what everyone else's opinion of me was and more certain of my own. Are you there yet? It can happen at any age, honey! It's a wonderful stage that I had no idea would come so soon or be so profound.

Radiating joy is easier because I'm not hiding behind presumptions and manipulations to get others to either like me or do what I want them to do. There's a certainty of knowing my purpose in life, believing I was created for that purpose, feeling confident in my marriage and my parenting, and having some sense of executive credibility in my area of expertise. Heck, I'm even pretty good at gardening, cooking, entertaining, party planning, home decorating, and packing for a trip to the Big Apple in one carry-on bag!

And while I can now fly with just a single well-stuffed carry-on, I can assure you that learning to like myself was a real road trip, one that revealed a lot about my relationships with others. If you're heading this way, drive carefully; I've left a lot of baggage on the roads. It wasn't as if I went to bed and while I slept off my remaining hours as a thirty-nine-year old it all changed.

> *"Your relationship with others is a mirror*
> *of your relationship with yourself."*
>
> —Mitzi Purdue

I am one of those who needed to work on a relationship with myself. It's always easier to be "on stage" with others if your personality is one full of drama. Part of learning to be comfortable with being alone is that it requires you to deal with yourself, talk to yourself, look at yourself, and answer the questions in your head. I suppose it's why a lot of sanguine types don't like being alone. Liking yourself starts with being honest with yourself about your true intentions, desires, motives, and ultimately what you believe you were called to do. And then you have to answer that calling.

PPF's

For me, answering that calling required a little self-image surgery on my attitude toward my appearance. The attention I gave to outward appearance created a disorder that I am going to call the "**P**hysical **P**henomena **F**lakes." It began with the first glance in the mirror at a very young age when I discovered that I in no way resembled the extraordinary beauties in the books I was reading, such as Belle, Snow White, or Cinderella. The flakes would come and go in mild to severe cases and could flare up due to a variety of things: taking an innocent comment the wrong way, feeling bloated during "that" time of the month, a friend not saving a seat for me at the lunch table . . . You get the point, and you can probably write your own list. As I moved into high school and beyond, the flakes accumulated like snowdrifts, creating obstacles that I allowed to become personal limitations.

As I've matured into adulthood and gained a perspective on those obstacles, I knew I wanted to help others struggling to overcome their own flakes and show them how to plow through their own snowdrifts. Although I didn't realize it in my younger years, I wasn't alone; others were going through the same thing. Who knew! If you're feeling the way I did, trust me when I say that you aren't the only one out there. That kind of thinking kept me from turning what I perceived to be obstacles into opportunities for growth, kept me from standing up to the questions that held me back, and kept me from being plain honest. When you create a lie that makes you feel better or believe one that a guy is telling you just so he can get what he wants, your self-respect withers. And I bet that right now, you're rolling some self-doubt questions around in your own heart and mind. Girl, I'm on that journey, too—see? I'm still not alone. And neither are you.

IT'S A JOURNEY

Part of the journey in writing this book included confronting many personal limitations and overcoming them. They took the form of questions I asked myself: "Who do you think you are? Why would someone want to read anything you have to say? What makes you so special?" Well, I'm certainly not any more special than anyone else. Actually I'm very much like a lot of other experts and authors. We all decided we simply could NOT keep quiet with "our" story, and because it is ours, it's unique. As I have embraced my own exclusive container, gifts, talents, and style over the years, I recognized that I was my toughest critic. For years, I focused on perfection, which turned out to be a very limiting goal. Part of the magic of turning forty—of getting comfortable in my own skin— was realizing the value of a new goal: excellence instead of perfection. "Being a true human BEcoming" is a phrase that helps me focus on being proactive, as opposed to just a human "being." As Benjamin Franklin said, "Hide your talent not, for greatness you were made; what good is a sundial if left in the shade?"

Whether it's self-inflicted or instigated by others, please know that this blistering PPF syndrome is mainly controlled by your own thinking. It metastasizes by keeping your attention on one side or the other—the inside or the outside—sabotaging the precarious balance we need. Both extremes present an unhealthy approach to beauty: the neglectful one and the narcissistic one. As one incredible lady put it to me recently, "Possibly the biggest miss in blending inner and outer beauty is that we don't pay enough attention to the second part of the second-greatest commandment: love your neighbor **as yourself**! You simply cannot love others well without first loving yourself."

Wise words indeed from Mitzi Purdue, widow of the late Frank Purdue of Purdue Chicken and daughter of Sheraton Hotel founder Ernest Flagg Henderson. I had a unique opportunity to interview her on some of these very issues. It was such an exceptional moment for me that it was as if we were drinking a cup of tea at a quaint café in Manhattan. That's just the kind of woman she is—exceptional. She says that "investing in beauty is a great idea and very worth it at any age or stage of life. It will absolutely energize you and improve your relationships with others."

And this takes effort. Mitzi agrees that personal grooming takes energy, and oftentimes, it takes help, so honey, go get some! "Whether it's through a trusted friend or a hired professional, everyone benefits from the results of that collaboration because you will put your best foot forward." She shared a story of how she recently had a friend come over to take pictures of her dressed in approximately thirty-five of her best "go-to" outfits, complete with earrings, shoes, hose, all accessories, and a purse. She then created a board with these outfits on them that hangs just inside her closet. (And, boy, would I love to go in that closet!) The time she says it saves her when she has an important luncheon, dinner party, or meeting to dress for is invaluable. "All I have to do is look at the picture board, and I can find the most appropriate outfit in a snap."

Mitzi's strategy eliminates much of the frustration we often feel when trying to prepare our "container" for an event and in so doing enables her to stay focused on how her "contents" can be a blessing to others. Another benefit is how it minimizes the drama and time wasted in daily dressing and undressing and redressing. I think this is a brilliant idea that many women should employ. (**Author's note: Send me a picture of your "Naked to Knockout Go-to Style Board" at wendy@wendylynonline. com and you'll receive a special gift. Include the picture in your e-mail for posting on my Web site, wendylynonline.com.**)

Mitzi herself is an author. In her book *I Didn't Bargain for This!* she has chronicled her life story from very early childhood and upbringing to the death of the love of her life and even now . . . life after. It is an amusing read full of life's challenges, her travels abroad, and what her life was like growing up. The Hendersons put a premium on hard work, family values, education, and contributing to society. Mitzi did all of that and remained grounded; oozed with optimism; and displayed kindness, resourcefulness, gracefulness, empathy, and, yes, beauty on the inside AND out!

Another woman who offers some great insight on the topic of living balanced lives is author Lisa Bloom. In her book *Think*, she challenges us to take ownership of the power we have to think for ourselves. In refer-ring to the unbalanced lives of women, Lisa sends a wake-up call to help us get back on track. "The first step is to reclaim time in our lives. We are overwhelmingly exhausted, running ourselves ragged with the work, housework, kids, laundry, repeat, repeat. Women say, 'I don't ever have time to think. All I can do is watch *Real Housewives* at the end of the day. I don't have the mental space for anything else.' Not true. The second step is to read: read more, read serious articles, serious journalism and most of all read books. Eighty percent of Americans didn't read one book last year. The third step is not letting other people tell you what to do or think. Stop listening to blowhards and experts. I want women to think for themselves, to do research on what's important to them. We have unprecedented access to information; almost all of us can go to **Google** and get credible, authoritative answers to the questions in our lives. We should be doing that, not listening to others. Lastly, reconnect and engage with the world around you. Find out what's going on in your community: Is the library in danger of closing? Does the battered women's shelter need help?"

Your ability to think in healthy ways and walk securely in your worth holds the key to a successful princess story ending, whether you see a Sleeping Beauty in the mirror or not . . . And who knows, maybe she's just sleeping. The world needs you. Check your pulse; if you're still breathing, then there's a purpose for your being here! Next time you get stalled on your journey to being sexy in your own skin, listen closely. Are you hear-ing the same questions I was? "Who do you think you are? What makes you so special?" The louder the questions seem to sound, the closer you probably are to freeing yourself from everyone else's opinions. And if you need just a little boost, here are the right answers to those questions: "I'm special because I'm me, and God didn't have time to create a nobody—just a somebody.

Your life is a gift . . . What you do with your life is the gift you give back.

There's no doubt the cost is high for the woman who lives her whole life chasing after what others define as true beauty. "Pretty" is a fact we can all comment on while "beauty" is a force to be reckoned with. Beauty through the seasons and at all ages of life takes on many forms . . . the confidence these women exhibit however, is quite similar. At some point, we have to quit the striving and just "be." I think this description of our seasons of life puts it well and helps us all get perspective. I'm sure you can relate . . . .

WHEN A WOMAN LOOKS IN THE MIRROR

Age 3: She looks at herself and sees a queen! "I am beautiful."

Age 8: She looks at herself and sees herself as Cinderella or Sleeping Beauty. "I *think* I'm beautiful."

Age 15: She looks at herself and sees herself as the "know-it-all" Cinderella or cheerleader, or if she is PMSing, she sees fat . . . pimples . . . UGLY. ("Mom, I can't go to school looking like this!")

Age 20: She looks at herself and sees "too fat/too thin," "too short/too tall," "too straight/too curly"—but decides she's going anyway. "I have other qualities that will make up for it."

Age 30: She rarely has time to look at herself, but when she does, sees "too fat/too thin," "too short/too tall," "too straight/too curly"—but decides she doesn't have time to fix herself, so she fixes the kids to look cute and she goes anyway.

Age 40: She looks at herself and sees "too fat/too thin," "too short/too tall," "too straight/too curly"—but says "At least I'm clean" and goes forth. But unless her glasses are on, sometimes she doesn't see close enough to be objective anyway.

Age 50: She looks at herself and sees "I am" and goes wherever she wants to go.

Age 60: She looks at herself and reminds herself of all the people who can't even see themselves in the mirror anymore. She goes out and conquers the world.

Age 70: She looks at herself and sees wisdom, laughter, and talent and then goes out and enjoys life.

Age 80: She doesn't bother to look. She just puts on a purple hat and figures, "As long as I can still go, I'm going out to have fun with the world."

Regardless of your age when you take the glance, being able to catch the lie that's speaking back from the mirror is something we may have to face our whole lives through. I encourage you to find the funny, engage in being empowering through self-talk, and be true to yourself. One way to feel sexy in your own skin is to acknowledge that change is inevitable. With quantity of years comes great quality of life, or at least a more balanced perspective. No matter how much we want to deny it, our containers are withering away, and what's left to last is what's in them.

What about You?

Women at every age have used their bodies, their dress (or lack thereof), their appeal, and their power since the beginning of time. I think of the incredible legacy of women in the Old and New Testaments who used theirs for both good and not-so-good results. Ruth, Delilah, Esther, Mary, Deborah, and, of course, Eve: there are countless others, and what's worth noting is the obvious fact that man has had an obsession with appearance and used women for gain because of it since the foundation of time. We can learn from history about how to use our physical prowess significantly rather than flamboyantly.

Then there are the more recent world shapers such as Mary Kay Ash, Oprah Winfrey, Helen Keller, Betsy Ross, Anne Frank, Rosa Parks, Kay Arthur, Amy Grant, Sarah Palin, Geraldine Ferraro, Condoleezza Rice, Joyce Meyer, and Beth Moore. These women have used their containers to reshape the world for those they served. It's no wonder that a common bond of these great leaders was to use their influence for a common good. They thought courageously enough to be the change and acted boldly enough to announce that change would be worth it. They used their own special megaphones to get their points across. Brilliant salespeople! Their charm, character, and self-confidence led them to be pillars in history. Why not you? What special gift, talent, cause, or mission can you begin or even follow through with?

So, you see, using your body as a tool for selling isn't altogether a bad thing. We're all selling something . . . . It might seem like all you're

selling is the benefit of getting your children to believe that eating car-
rots really means they'll be able to see in the dark. If so, do it with gusto;
you're an example of an everyday saleswoman doing a worthy job. You
may be landing million-dollar deals or speaking for thousands of dollars.
Whatever your product, please remember that the first thing you sell is
YOU. When you don't, you're still selling—you're selling yourself a lie
that you're not worth it. Such a mind-set can unravel your world one lie,
one day at a time.

The depth of depression and ruin that the road of pride can take you
on is horrendous, as we will see in some of the women's stories that I've
included in this book. And, yes, pride has two sides: thinking of yourself
more highly than you should and also thinking too lowly of yourself.
Most women exhibit pride on one faulty level or another, and we can all
do a better job of teaching our daughters how to balance the scale. If you
don't have daughters, don't worry. There's always another woman nearby
who needs an example to follow. For me, being both the student and the
teacher has been rewarding.

TRIBUTE TO MARY KAY ASH

I've been mentored by many whom I am fortunate enough to be considered a "daughter" of, and none has made a more profound impact
than Mary Kay Ash. Her life exemplified the essence of inner and outer
beauty. Her tough and tender approach to life's obstacles makes her a role
model still today. Most know her for being a makeup mogul; I knew her
for being a "Go-Give" and Golden Rule implementer. She sold hope for a
better way of life more than she sold lipstick. She sold self-esteem to her
sales force because she had it in her container to pass on. Her definition
of happiness was having something to do that you love to do, someone to
love, and something to look forward to. I couldn't agree more with that
prescription for a balanced and happy life. Mary Kay was most noted
for her integrity in leadership. She says, *"I put a lot of emphasis on how
to treat people. The reason for this is simple. The real success of our
personal lives and careers can best be measured by the relationships we*

have with the people most dear to us—our family, friends, and cowork-ers. If we fail in this aspect of our lives, no matter how vast our worldly possessions or how high on the corporate ladder we climb, we will have achieved very little." She's the kind of leader I believe we can all be inspired to emulate. Her core principles and balanced ego caused her to be a true beauty, but even more, she followed the priorities she preached. When a caliber of woman like that finds a way to merge what's on her inside with a sense of class and style on the outside, you have the essence of a knockout!

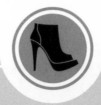

STEP UP TO ACTION:
Rewind and Rewire

Yes, the negative self-doubt tapes still continue at times to play back in the Wendy Lyn tape player of life. I have to rewind and rewire sometimes, and maybe you do, too! How? Try asking yourself these questions:

Have I used positive self-talk effectively to rewire my thoughts when needed?

Am I celebrating the less frequent occurrences of negative self-talk?

Have I made myself accountable to anyone? There's strength in numbers! Do I ask for help? Do I balance my independence with involvement from others? What areas might I be overly co-dependent in?

What one thing can I do to celebrate being comfortable in my own skin?

Chapter 3

BEAUTY AND THE BEAST

"Our deepest fear is not that we are inadequate. Our deepest fear is that we are powerful beyond measure. It is our light, not our darkness that most frightens us. We ask ourselves, who am I to be brilliant, gorgeous, talented, and fabulous? Actually, who are you not to be? You are a child of God.

Your playing small does not serve the world. There is nothing enlightened about shrinking so that other people won't feel insecure around you. We are all meant to shine, as children do. We were born to make manifest the glory of God that is within us. It's not just in some of us; it's in all of us. And as we let our own light shine, we unconsciously give other people permission to do the same. As we are liberated from our own fear, our presence automatically liberates others."

—Nelson Mandela

I love that quote because I can relate to it. "Your playing small does not serve the world." A small mentality will not expand to greatness. Thinking BIG . . . now that's a pathway to a giant impact. Another benefit of being comfortable in your own skin is that it propels you on your mission. It helps you embrace the possibility of "what if . . . ," and when that happens, you truly become a catalyst for change . . . giving permission for others to soar . . . paving roadways in the desert. There is beauty in serving your fellow man.

How quickly, though, we can move from a beauty model to a beastly one. Don't you know some Jekyll-and-Hyde people? One minute they are full of compliments and affirmations, and the next, they are manipulating you for their gain. And even though you know what's happening, they are so good at it that you give in anyway. The finesse used for sordid gain will often turn any beauty one does possess to an ugly, beastly aura in a flash.

We all have a tendency to act more beastly when we're tired, hungry, deprived, or disappointed. That sounds like every mother of a newborn, a two-year-old, or a teenager; a menopausal woman; a working mom . . . yep, just about every one of you, right? When the monster of unmet expectations, selfish living, and ungodly speech dares to come out of you, remember that we've all been there. There's both forgiveness when you blow it and discipline to withstand the urge; it just depends on what part of the circle you're on. More experiences of blowing it usually help you decide you don't want to repeat it . . . again!

Why is it that this happens so naturally, so frequently, so like every day between moms and teenage daughters? Apart from the scientific approach to dismiss the actions based on emotional estrogen, I can tell you I dread those days coming between my daughters and me. My bet is that my prayer life will increase and my knees will get more of a workout. In *Bringing up Girls,* Dr. James Dobson states that the disconnect experienced between mothers and daughters who are between the ages of thirteen and eighteen happens when attachment during the early stages of life was neglected. It has been demonstrated further that the failure of mothers and babies to attach is linked directly to all types of physical and mental illnesses. The reason is apparent. If a child is regularly overwhelmed by negative feelings and stressful circumstances, his or her inability to cope in infancy becomes a lifelong pattern. The link between maternal attachment and poor health is not merely theoretical; it is reality (*Bringing up Girls,* page 61). This is most often why mothers and daughters disconnect. When they do and how severely the consequences are can be enormous and even life threatening.

YOUNG WOMEN NEED ROLE MODELS

Why am I bringing up a topic like this? Because every woman reading this book, whether she has daughters or not, can have a significant impact on the young women growing up around her. That includes you. You may be an aunt, a neighbor, a teacher, a community volunteer, or a business professional whom others look up to. The choice you make to look in the mirror and like what you see can eliminate (or at least minimize) your negative feelings about yourself; having a healthy self-image strengthens your ability to deal with stressful circumstances. Added together, those two things can build a healthy pattern for your daughter (and other women around you) to follow. Your choice not to play small, as Mr. Mandela so eloquently put it, allows your own light to shine, liberating you from your own fear and liberating others in the process.

LET YOUR LIGHT SHINE

How can you be an influence? It starts with knowing who you are and being comfortable in your own skin, as we discussed in the prior chapter. The way you view and value yourself is rooted in your own upbringing; by giving others the power to define who you are, you inadvertently communicate that you are only as "valuable" or "worthy" as someone else's opinion. And opinions change faster than the price of oil, don't they? Needing a higher beauty approval rating from the public or the media will always be unsatisfying because it's a moving target; even if we hit it one day, it changes the next, and something inside of us is continually empty and unhappy and . . . well, beastly. If you are one of the eighty-three percent of women who are unhappy with their body image, you likely look in the mirror and on some level see or hear the beast rather than the beauty that you have to offer. And whether you realize it or not, that image that you "see" is what you are communicating to the next generation of young women. Will you be a hindrance to their self-image obstacles or a help to their seeing the opportunities that await? Will you play small or choose to let your light shine?

This isn't just a call to mothers of young daughters. Whether you have sons, grown daughters, or no children at all, Dr. Dobson is raising the flag of awareness over this need for younger women to have the positive influence of a mother figure if they are to have a healthy self-image. And sometimes, the consequences of that missing mother can be very painful for a tweenager. When you have to ask an adult to help you go pick out your first bra or mention that you think you need deodorant, it can be damaging to your self-esteem. These are milestones to be celebrated, not dreadful, embarrassing events to be avoided! And you can't avoid them, anyway; they are simply part of a young girl's journey to womanhood.

WHEN THE JOURNEY GETS BUMPY

Meet my friend Ruthie.

This is her story. Her mother was present . . . well, kinda . . . but becoming increasingly sick. As the years flew by, her mother's health flew away, thanks to a diagnosis of MS. Her deterioration seemed to pick up speed such that she could no longer care for herself, much less two kids and a husband. Ruth's father had a prominent job as a pastor and head-master of a large college. He traveled a lot because he was sought after for speaking engagements, which meant the family was often on their own. He didn't intend to forsake the family at all; he loved them and thought he was working hard at providing for them. As the medical bills piled up, so did the stress. And while neither parent abandoned the family liter-ally, what did get abandoned was Ruthie's need for a maternal figure and strong communication during these very formative years.

Left with no one to talk to about her inner struggles, questions about maturity, concern over her mother's deterioration, and even questions about God, Ruthie sought to find answers in secret corners, closets, and the solace of her small room. When the pressure and frustration were too great, she would make a small cut on her inner arm and feel a sense of release. . . . Ahh, finally something she could control. The powerful way it began to make her feel better was an unfortunate affirmation to do it again. So she did. The road of self-mutilation overtook Ruthie for about three years, all without her parents or friends knowing about it. The secrets that the walls in a home hold . . . if only they could speak. Then again, most of us probably wouldn't want to know . . . or maybe we would all find out how very similar we are. What you do in secret is a powerful thing. Beginning to devalue her body by cutting it opened the door for Ruth to lower her personal property price tag. Her own value began to decline. She became vulnerable and gave in. One poor choice led to another, and at fifteen, she found herself pregnant and dealing with guilt and shame for eight full months as she continued to keep her new secret "private."

Unfortunately, there is always a consequence to our actions. Poor choices generally result in things working out poorly for us. Since her father was a leader in the community, not to mention under major stress with an ailing wife, Ruthie did not want to tell him. The truth is that no one knew except her boyfriend and a couple of confidential counselors at her school who gave her the "day-after pill" (which obviously failed) and who continued to counsel her toward abortion. Since she didn't show much and was such a good secret keeper, at eight months pregnant she even went on international travels with her father, and the family was still unaware. Ruth wasn't liking what she saw in the mirror but was beginning to realize the enormity of the fact that soon, two would be looking back.

Knowing that soon the truth would be common knowledge, even with her plan to give the child up for adoption, she would have to confess. Something strange had been going on inside Ruthie. It was beyond "growing" more than just a human life. SHE was indeed changing, in need of forgiveness and acceptance, and she found both in her earthly father and her heavenly father the day she revealed it all. With just weeks left to go before the baby would be born, Ruth ended her relationship with the boyfriend (a "poor choice" from the beginning) and sought out new friends who supported and better lined up with her belief systems as she pressed through a most difficult time. Her family loved and supported her as best they could, and to say it was an adjustment for them all is, well, an understatement.

LOVE WINS OUT

There is ONE who sees all our actions, public and private. He knows our thoughts, our intentions, our motives, and our secrets, and He loves us anyway. This is how your story can have a happy ending, too.

Today Ruth is a happily married mother of three, including her gift from heaven; she chose to keep her son, who is now twelve years old. The subject is still tender, but Ruth was courageous to share with me that LIFE is not a mistake; all life is to be valued. The decisions made in creating life earlier than desired carried big sacrifices for Ruthie—and anyone else, for that matter. Even if you think you CAN handle it, think again. Ruth raised her son during his first two years in a home with a mostly absent mother (mentally, physically, and emotionally), a mostly physically absent father, and a brother who was away at college; it was not the perfect setting for nightly feedings, crying, diaper changes, or a two-year-old's tantrums. But it didn't end there; it wasn't just the first two years. Babies grow and become toddlers . . . who become school aged . . . and now, who was going to marry a twenty-year-old gal with a four-year-old child?

The questions plagued Ruthie for what seemed an eternity. She worked on her inner character, learning to forgive herself and others. And she worked on the most important relationship of all, the one with her maker. She looked to God's word for some consolation and answers for her purpose in life. As a single mother, when you have a child depending on your survival skills, you tend to approach the obstacle or opportunity question a little more ferociously. When the dark clouds of life happen, they are often the precursor to a blue sky and rainbow just behind them. I, too, have had those cloudy times, ones that lingered and never disappeared with the wave of a magic wand. I have prayed through situations for others and even that situations in my own life would change. And when the circumstance didn't change, I did.

In Ruth's story, we see a beautiful example of new life, one emerging literally and the other spiritually. As a strong and more confident woman, wife, and mother today, Ruthie says she never wants to go back through that time, but she wouldn't change it because of who she's become in the process. Ruthie chose "not to play small" because it served no one—not her, not her son, not the world. Her choices to grow through her obstacles have tamed the beast that wanted to destroy her beauty. In this beautiful story, it's love that won.

What about you? Do you fight and even flee when the clouds come? Is confrontation your invitation to exit the party? Are you "outta here"? If so, I encourage you to ask these three questions when the clouds are closing in:

• What's good about this?

• What can I learn from this?

• What can I do to change it?

If the beast is always hovering, if the urge to fight or flee feels like your only choice, then I would encourage you to seek help sooner rather than later. Whether your struggles are played out through sexual behaviors, drug and alcohol addictions, self-mutilation, excessive partying, or isolation, know that any bad habit taken to the extreme (or sometimes any good habit taken to the extreme) needs acknowledgment. Admitting where you are so you are able to navigate where you want to go is the first step to any positive change. Ultimate help comes from someone greater than you. The only higher being able to take the ugly, miry clay and turn it into something beautiful is the Lord Jesus Christ. It's His job to mold and create, and He is certainly still in the miracle-working business! Gospel music giant Mandisa sings it straight up: "When the waves are taking you under, hold on just a little while longer. This is gonna make you stronger, stronger."

My finite vision reminds me of my big picture limitations. What happens "to me" if often happening "for me" . . . for me to learn, grow, make adjustments, and pass on the lesson. It's about so much more than just me! There's more than me who needs a dose of healthy self-esteem: it's the children God has entrusted us with to will be an example that will help prepare them for life. It's your extended family, your community network, your circle of influence that will benefit from your valuable life lessons passed along. Some are drowning and need a lifesaver thrown out – YOU just might be the person to toss it. Leaving a legacy for the next generation can be part of what gives your life purpose. Our perspective to pay it forward creates a beautiful future for the recipients we may never even know. When I finally gave birth to my daughters, I instantly knew I would be forever changed, as was Cindy, who wrote this beautiful poem.

The Love of a Mother

When I was just a daughter, I really couldn't see it.
Now I am a mom and I can hardly conceive it.
The love for a daughter is love like no other.
I'm trying to comprehend this love of a mother.

It happened so quickly and now it is so clear,
looking at my daughter's face and feeling her so near.
There was my baby girl looking up at me,
the world was standing still and I could finally see.
My life had changed forever: I knew this to be true
God said "Here's your princess I created just for you."

Wanting her to grow or not . . . Oh, it tears me apart,
this love for my daughter is so real in my heart.
Her bright eyes, her precious smile . . . go with me every day,
If she's not beside me, she's never far away.
We've cried and laughed together when no one else was there.
This bond that's been created is one we'll always share.

My daughter's a young woman now, it cannot be denied.
One day she will marry and he'll be at her side.
Soon she'll have a little girl and she will feel this love.
When she sees that precious face, she'll thank God above.
Her life will forever change: I know this to be true
She's not just a daughter now; a Mom has been born too.

Yes, when I was just a daughter, I really could not see it.
Now I am a Mom and I know that I can feel it.
This love for a daughter is love like no other
I finally comprehend this love of a Mother.

By Cindy E. Becerra

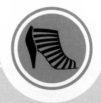

STEP UP TO ACTION:

Liberated to Leave a Legacy

Is there an area where your playing small is hindering you from moving forward?

What typically triggers a "beastly" metamorphosis in you?

How can you steer clear in advance?

List the names of some young women you now have (or could have) a direct influence on. For whom can you be a mentor to?

To find out more about making improvements inside and out, take the free assessment at www.NakedtoKnockout.com and click on Word2Wendy

Chapter 4

MIRROR, MIRROR
ON THE WALL . . .

My first year cheerleading was in sixth grade. I remember the feeling of wearing my uniform for the first time and looking in the mirror and thinking I had arrived. My father was in the military at the time, and we had just returned from a three-year stay in the Netherlands. I spoke fluent Dutch and German because we always lived in the communities with the locals, not on a base. While I loved the multicultural friends I had gained from attending an international school, I was really excited to be Americanized again and enjoy the simple pleasures such as apple pie, skateboarding, learning how to use a curling iron on my own hair, French fries as opposed to "frites," hot dogs as opposed to "wurst," the Bee Gees, softball, and, yes, my new love: cheerleading. I loved that uniform! The only problem with the cute skirt and top was that my legs were very skinny and my chest was very flat. Other girls seemed to be budding while I was just boney. Looking back at that mirror moment when I thought I'd arrived, well, what I'd really arrived at was a frustration with the way I looked compared with all the other girls on the squad. It was easy to compare my lack with their reward. Excelling in gymnastics gave me an edge to stand out and seemed to make up for some of my deficit in the personal appearance arena. *My takeaway: find something you can do well and focus on improving what you can control, not dwelling on what you can't.*

What happens when women look in the mirror is this: "Oh, gracious, do I really look like that?" Our thoughts snowball downhill: "Crap, I *used* to look waaay better!" until we end up at "When did this happen?

Growing old just plain sucks sometimes. I guess I have other qualities . . . but I'm really starting to look like my mother!"

No matter how many beneficial reasons (such as pregnancy and childbirth) I come up with for the spider veins and skin discoloration, it doesn't make them less noticeable or welcomed. So sometimes I cover them up with body bronzer. Sometimes I act like it doesn't matter and refuse to notice them. And then sometimes the reflection just jumps off the mirror yelling, "Imperfections! Flaws! Blemishes! Gross!"

Doesn't that happen to you? Come on; be honest. I know I'm not the only one talking so ugly to myself about myself. (It's really worse, but I'm taming my quotes for print—Ha!) And I know I'm not the only one who has to work at using healthy self-talk. Consistent, disciplined doses of healthy self-talk make all the difference. It's mental conditioning, and like a physical muscle, mental toughness can be developed and strengthened with practice. Here is where the power of choice comes into play and, with it, the domino effect. How I choose to react leads either to results that prosper me or to the pantry for another bag of M&M's. For other women, however, this cycle can end in a trench called abuse, neglect, and addictions that lead to all kinds of eating, sleeping, and personality disorders. If you are prone to wander into such a trench, STOP, put this book down, and get help immediately. There are many referral services printed in the back of this book, along with national Web sites for you to use. When in doubt about what to do, ask a trusted friend to assist you in finding the help you need.

THE REALITY IS . . .

These unhealthy reactions are often driven by our interpretation of the image we see in the mirror, an interpretation based on how we compare what we are seeing to the magazine covers, movie close-ups, and media mayhem. And in our mirror, we inevitably fall short.

The problem is the mirror isn't lying to us; the magazine covers are. The beauty industry is famous for airbrushing techniques, using all the latest tricks for making skin look perfect. The touch-ups are endless.

Hair is done by a stylist right before the shoot, and someone else has ironed and selected all the clothes. And we are taught to buy the notion that people in Hollywood actually look like this in everyday life. In 2002, actress Jamie Lee Curtis decided she'd had enough of all that and set off quite a fracas when she had *More* magazine do a no-holds-barred before-and-after photo shoot of her. Yes, before all the pro staffers went to work and then, three hours and thirteen staffers later, the after. The then-44-year-old actress wanted to emphasize that even high-profile celebrities look "normal" without the help of a team of makeup artists and digital alterations.

The buzz that Jamie Lee's article created didn't last long, and nothing has really changed. The culture still peddles two equally ridiculous scenarios: one is that you can look like Barbie every day—if you have enough money to hire all the right people with all the right tools; the other is that, with enough surgery, you can morph your body into different shapes that you believe to be more visually appealing.

I have to stop right here and say that while the entire rest of my book is about using skin care, makeup, clothes, the right hairstyle, and jewelry to properly adorn yourself to the max, I do believe that there is a limit. Women should not fall victim to the media obsession with physical beauty. A recent poll indicated that girls on college campuses knew the names of the Kardashians but could not quote the names of wars we were currently in. How sad that the names and images of women who don't live in the real world have become more important than the real world.

I hope I have been really clear that a focus on inner beauty and character first can be a powerful prerequisite to bringing out our physical best. Once you have a foundation of who you are and who you are unwilling to compromise yourself to be, your quest to be your best self on the outside can flourish. If you need a brow or eye lift, a neck lift, or any other enhancement and it is something you have discussed with the people in your life who matter most, then go for it. And if Spanx aren't enough, then add that area to the fixer-upper list as well. We put holes in our ears where there were none. We add jewelry to parts of our body besides our earlobes. We take permanent ink and tattoo graphics on our body. We dye our hair all sorts of colors; we even add fake hair for extensions and fullness. We put on fake nail tips, eyelashes, and tans, and it seems the saga never ends. A few of my clients have had really good results with permanent makeup, which is yet another beauty issue to address. If you're all about being current, you'll find yourself wearing platform shoes to appear taller and in style. Even men can add a lift to their shoes for added height. There are endless ways to "step up" your outer shell with class. We'll all benefit from giving the barn a good coat of paint, if that's what it needs.

Careful, though: all this fascination with enhancements can easily suck you into the abyss of "never enough." It's what I call the cotton candy syndrome. At first glance, cotton candy not only is super visually enticing but also creates a mental appeal. As your taste buds begin to water and your hand lifts the fluffy substance closer to your mouth, your anticipation heightens, and then, poof! You get the pink cloudlike candy inside your mouth to enjoy, and before you can even swirl it around with your tongue, it's gone, over, down the esophagus. The whole experience is totally over in ten seconds or less. It simply doesn't fulfill. Not all physical "updates" present exactly this same scenario, but they can. Turning yourself into eye candy at the expense of your inner character is a recipe for heartache, wallet ache, and more. I am simply sounding a warning to alert the check-and-balance part of your ego that is brilliant enough without all the add-ons to deal with. Here's another story to prove my point.

KILLER SECRETS

We've all seen the scenario where beauty queens go to unbelievable ends as they strive for perfection. The cost of losing that title pushes them to be satisfied only with winning. And they do it on a body that is already perfect by most of the public's opinion. Can the mirror really lie that poorly? Can a woman be driven to such desperate means that she turns to horrible, life-threatening addictions?

In Allison's life, it was all true. And just before the ball of yarn started unraveling for her, seemingly incredible and wonderful things were happening. She was at the top of her life, an A+ student as a freshman in high school, the national baton-twirling and dance titles were within reach, and as an only child, she was deeply loved by both parents.

So how does a beautiful young girl with all this going for her end up with a toilet bowl as her best friend for the next three years? It's a question we all wonder about, and it's a question I investigated. When I interviewed Allison Kreiger Walsh, Miss Florida 2006, she was very candid and open to sharing all she could to increase awareness of eating disorders and to help even one young gal or mother expose their struggle. Allison is now healed and is doing the best thing possible. She's keeping the flame burning with a bright light these days. Her radiance is now an obvious one that burns from within. Her confidence is not dependent on the outcome of a "performance," another's strict critique, a score, or even what she sees in the mirror alone. It's an all-encompassing formula of being certain of who you are from the inside out. And she's winning with finesse.

Before heading off to the University of Florida, Allison shared her secret with her parents and sought out treatment. She knew that if she didn't get help, she might not make it to college. How bad was it? "I was both bulimic and anorexic. I was a perfect secret keeper; I knew all the private places to do what I needed to do to get my quick fixes daily. I would binge and purge sometimes seven times a day. I had been doing this for three years before it got so bad that I simply couldn't deal with the stress anymore. Not even my boyfriend knew. When I told my parents, they were in denial and shock for the first month or so. Then they knew, too, that I had to get help. So my entire senior year I worked with treatment specialists: a psychiatrist, a psychologist, and a dietician all helping me learn how to eat healthily. They told me that college campuses were a breeding ground for this kind of behavior and that I needed to totally heal, get accountable, and make strong changes or I would either fall into other bad habits or do this again and die. The choice was easy for me.

I'm a fighter." Giving up or lying down to die has never been an option for this competitive gal!

Allison did go to the University of Florida and earned her first title as a beauty queen: Miss U of F. Since this was a preliminary to the Miss Florida pageant, she qualified to compete. It took three years of grooming and determination, but eventually, in 2006, Allison Kreiger became Miss Florida! It represented so much more to Allison than a beauty queen title, though. To her, it provided a platform to get her message out about eating disorders and what needs to be done to help. In the process, she formed a nonprofit called H.O.P.E., for "Help Other People Eat." You can find out more at the Web site listed in this book's reference guide. Allison's message for you or someone you know who is a victim of any eating disorder is to seek out help immediately. Admit that it's a disease and know you're not alone. Recognize how out of balance your view of yourself is. Consider the long-term effects and decide that you are worth more than the hold it has on you. ***To live a beautiful life, you simply must be balanced, and taking care of yourself is a beautiful thing!***

If you suspect any of these symptoms in a friend, approach her in the most nonconfrontational manner possible. Point out the qualities that concern you and offer your support. Never mention body appearance or shape, as this becomes only more validating and encourages the poor behavior. You might want to say something like, "I noticed your endurance is lacking" or "I'm concerned about your health; are you getting enough sleep?" Women with beautiful bodies at every age struggle with appearance, acceptance, and association. I'm not sure it ever ends. One great way to diminish the pressure from others and live a life of purpose and peace is to agree with what God says about you. The Scriptures speak so clearly about how we can deal with our shell and clothe it without worrying about it in Matthew, chapter 6. Seeking God's ways aren't always the popular ways, but they are the ways that produce lasting, peaceful, and fulfilling results.

"Take time each day to prepare yourself so that you can present your best self to others. This will do wonders to increase your self-confidence."

—Allison Kreiger Walsh

Facts about Eating Disorders

- Bulimia, anorexia, and binge-eating disorders affect up to 24 million Americans and 70 million individuals worldwide, and they are the third most common chronic illness among adolescents.
- The risk of developing an eating disorder is 50%–80% genetic.
- Forty-two percent of first-grade through third-grade girls want to be thinner, and 81% of ten-year-olds are afraid of being fat.
- Eighty percent of all children have been on a diet by the time they have reached the fourth grade.
- One out of four people who are battling an eating disorder is male.
- Up to 19% of college-aged women in America are bulimic.
- Twenty to twenty-five percent of "normal dieters" progress to partial- or full-syndrome eating disorders.
- At least 50,000 individuals will die as a direct result of an eating disorder this year.
- One out of every ten victims of anorexia will die from side effects accompanying anorexia.
- Eating disorders usually affect teens, but the age is changing significantly; the number of children as young as seven and the number of women over fifty being treated have significantly increased in the past five years.

Surprised? I was, too. And that's part of the problem; most of us really don't understand these disorders or the needs that drive them because the victims are so good at keeping secrets. According to Dr. Zaid Malik,

a Little Rock, Arkansas, psychiatrist, "Eating disorder behavior is fulfilling some kind of need." Dr. Malik oversees the Eating Disorders Clinic
at the Psychiatric Research Institute of the University of Arkansas for
Medical Sciences. "Getting help early is the key to a patient getting her
life back on track."

And that's just what Allison's organization and its sister program, Get
R.E.A.L., Realistic Expectations and Attitudes for Life, are trying to do.
Get R.E.A.L. focuses on enhancing self-esteem, promoting a positive
body image, and preventing eating disorders from happening in the first
place. Both H.O.P.E. and Get R.E.A.L. are zeroing in on reaching young
people as soon as possible so that they can avoid some of the issues that
Dr. Malik and others like him see. They encourage people to get back
to the basics of taking care of themselves, to interpret media messages
appropriately, and to embrace overall wellness. Allison is working hard
to provide all age groups with the tools necessary to ensure a healthy
lifestyle, to eliminate dangerously unattainable and unrealistic standards,
and to develop a healthy response when they stand in front of the looking
glass and ask, "Mirror, mirror on the wall . . . ," whether they are wearing
a cheerleading uniform, a business suit, or nothing at all!

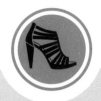

STEP UP TO ACTION:

Playing the Comparison Game Makes You a Loser Every Time

When do you find you are the most unconscious about your eating choices (as in "oblivious to caloric intake, their horrendous ingredients, and draining results")?

Is there an unhealthy cycle you see developing . . . daily, weekly, monthly?

Are you happy with your current body shape and workout program?

Is there someone you know who may have symptoms of anorexia or bulimia? If so, what are you willing to do about it?

List one healthy snack you want to start eating more of.

Check out the Web sites of Jillian Michaels and Suzanne Somers for awesome healthy recipes.

Chapter 5

CREATING COLOR CONFIDENCE

Never wear a red tie to an interview! If you haven't given that advice to someone, you should. Reading this chapter will help you know what color to wear to important events, interviews, or occasions and why. Color evokes emotion. Red is easy to relate to passion and anger when you consider how flushed your face gets from fits of rage, heightened blood pressure, and embarrassment. Wearing a red tie or blouse to an interview might leave the impression that you are simmering with anger. Not a good idea. While the effects of colors are mostly subliminal, like body language and other silent messages we send, giving attention to them can be very enjoyable and beneficial.

Customize your look with COLOR. It's the easiest way to spruce up some of what you already have in your wardrobe; It's a smart way to spruce up many of the neutral colors you probably have in your wardrobe; simply add a pop of color and "ta-da," you can go from drab to FAB. I especially think about what colors I'm wearing when it's raining and truly dreary outside. I want to be the sunshine when I enter a room, and color helps me remember to have a cheery disposition. Hey, some days, we all need a little reminding of that, don't we? Making a choice of what to wear on purpose is another disciplined effort you can make to be in better control of your emotions, rather than letting what you feel control your mood. Be proactive!

Understanding the meaning of certain colors can help you strategically select the right ones to wear. You can effectively set the right tone in your environment when you wear the appropriate colors. Choosing wisely creates a mood that can be highly advantageous in building your self-esteem and your relationships with others. Take note of the traditional banker: cool, calm, and collected blue. It's the color that conveys ultimate trustworthiness and respect. Purple has long been the color connected with royalty and mysticism, but it also implies sophistication and elegance. Maybe that's the reason the Purple Hat Society has chosen it as their brand mark.

WARM OR COOL?

It's happened to all of us. We've chosen the wrong color and don't even know it, until someone sincerely asks whether we're sick. If that's not bad enough, the wrong colors can also make us look older, heavier, and really tired. How can you choose correctly from so many hues? Sticking to some tried-and-true rules will help simplify it.

- Determine first whether your skin tone, eye color, and current hair color have stronger warm or cool color undertones. Do you see more blue in your skin tone (cool) or more gold, sallow, or olive (warm)? Once you know whether your skin has more yellow or blue undertones, you can build a wardrobe color scheme from there. Select colors within your color family to create various mix-and-match options.

- TEST: Hold a pure white piece of paper along with a manila file folder, which has a more creamy/beige hue, next to your face. See which one most introduces your face and complements it and which one competes with it for attention. For example, with the white paper, what do you see first, the paper or your face? The goal is to see YOU coming, not a loud, out-of-place color of fabric.

- Gold and silver jewelry can do the same trick, but most people like to wear both, so it isn't quite as good a test.

- Learn the meaning of colors and use them to your advantage, certainly as far as business dress is concerned. This is especially helpful during an interview and important presentations or selling appointments. Again, please refer to the chart for help.

• Don't rule out wearing colors that may not be your best; just don't wear them near your face!

Humans are very visually oriented; it's just the way we were made. Knowing how to make the most of color gives you a unique opportunity to affect others positively with what you wear daily. Getting a compliment on what you have on versus having someone ask you whether you're sick when, really, you're feeling fine is definitely one way to know how the color you're wearing is being received!

Wearing colors on purpose is a blessing to everyone. The rainbow gives us an example of how we feel when we see so many colors in one beautiful image. The colors combined with the natural wonder are an intriguing thing. It's also a gentle reminder of God's good promises. When he wanted something to be noticed and remembered, he used all the colors. Bold, loud—I like it! Use colors to get your message out in an effective and bold way, too.

COLOR CONFIDENCE

Nothing is more boring than plain beige worn up top and on your bottom. However, beige can be beautiful when coupled with a lace sweater, pearl jewelry, patent leather shoes, and a stunning red purse. Madonna is someone who can pull this look off with great style, complete with her signature red lipstick. For men, solid beige or tan pants are classic and can often be confidently worn with a black silk shirt or even a neatly pressed golf shirt. The fact that we're all different is part of what makes us unique. Allowing your true colors to be enjoyed and appreciated by others is one way to have an edge over your competition. Coloring outside the lines, having the courage to do it differently from how it's been done before, and adding in your own zest and spice will no doubt quickly help you stand out from the crowd. When your confidence and courage is strong enough to pull off a seemingly boring beige head to toe outfit and make it look totally classy and fab because you added one key accessory, like a bold red patent purse, you're on your way to stepping out in style. Another example is taking a navy pant and top and adding a kelly green purse, or opting for a glamour statement with gilded pieces—ie gold chain belt, jewelry or purse etc. You don't have to be Madonna to dress like a knockout!

Express yourself with color. Make use of the meanings of colors to project your desired impression.

Color	Meaning
RED:	warmth, love, anger, boldness, passion, speed, determination, courage
ORANGE:	cheerfulness, low cost, affordability, enthusiasm, stimulation, creativity
YELLOW:	attention grabbing, hunger, optimistic, comfort, liveliness, intellect, happiness, energy
GREEN:	reliability, luxurious, optimism, nature, calm, safety, honesty, optimism, harmony, freshness
BLUE:	peace, professionalism, loyalty, reliability, honor, melancholia, coldness
PURPLE:	power, royalty, elegance, sophistication, artificial, luxury, mystery, magic
GRAY:	conservatism, traditionalism, intelligence, serious, dull
BROWN:	relaxing, confident, casual, nature, solid, reliable, genuine, endurance
BLACK:	elegance, sophistication, formality, power, strength, depression, morbidity
WHITE:	cleanliness, purity, newness, peace, innocence, simplicity, sterility, snow

Using seasons of the year to capture particular color families that best suit an individual is a method that has been around for years. There's much talk about knowing what season your skin tone, hair, and eyes most resemble. How you use the information to your benefit can yield great rewards when you realize you are truly selling *you* even before you sell your products. In the business and political arena today, women do well to take note of small ways to boost their image and stand out. *I like to think of it as being "memorable."* Is your overall statement helping your audience (whether it's your family, your clients, a small presentation or networking event, or on stage as a professional speaker) REMEMBER YOU?

What follows is a list of some basics for the color theory. My premise has always been that every woman can wear almost every color, as long as she finds the right shade that naturally complements her. There are six criteria in all; first, determine whether warm or cool tones are best for you, and then consider from among deep, light, soft, or clear. To help you visualize these in real life, I've included a list of some celebrities you may relate to with certain color characteristics. After that, I've provided suggestions by season. See whether you can decide which of the six color families you fall into.

1. *Warm:* No cool undertones; think Reba McEntire or Sarah Ferguson

2. *Cool:* No warm undertones; think Christie Brinkley or Liz Hurley

3. *Clear:* Clear and bright; think Courteney Cox or a young Liz Taylor

4. *Soft:* Soft and muted; think Sarah Jessica Parker or Jennifer Aniston

5. *Light:* Light and delicate; think Gwyneth Paltrow or Heather Locklear

6. *Deep:* Dark and rich; think Cher or Kim Kardashian

The Four Seasons

WINTER colors are likened to the bright and clear jewel tones: magenta, pine green, burgundy, royal blue, pure white, true red, royal purple, and icy pink.

You will look best in WINTER (cool) colors if:

SKIN:

• Very white or white with slight pink tone

- Beige (not sallow)

- Gray-beige or brown

- Rosy

- Olive

- Black sallow or black/blue undertone

HAIR:

- Blue-black

- Dark brown (may have red highlights)

- Medium ash brown

- Salt and pepper, silver-gray

- White or white blond (rare)

EYES:

- Dark red-brown, black-brown

- Hazel (brown plus blue or green)

- Gray-blue, blue, or green, with white flecks in iris; may have gray rim

- Dark blue, violet

- Gray-green

JEWELRY:

- Silver tone is best

SPRING colors are likened to the light and muted pastels: bright coral, light moss, camel, denim, clear red, true green, and mango.
You will look best in SPRING (warm) colors if:

SKIN:

- Creamy ivory or ivory with golden freckles

- Peach or pink

- May have pink/purple knuckles

- Golden beige or golden brown

- Rosy cheeks (may blush easily)

HAIR:

- Flaxen blond

- Yellow or honey blond

- Strawberry blond or redhead (usually with freckles), auburn

- Golden brown or reddish black (rare)

- Dove gray or creamy white

EYES:

- Blue with white rays, clear blue, or steel blue

- Green with golden flecks, clear green

- Aqua or teal

- Golden brown

JEWELRY:

- Gold tone is best

SUMMER colors are likened to the paler versions of winter: lavender, raspberry, aqua, deep rose, cocoa, and soft fuchsia.
You will look best in SUMMER (cool) colors if:

SKIN:

- Pale beige with pink cheeks

- Beige with no cheek color, even sallow

- Rosy beige or rosy brown; very pink

- Gray brown

HAIR:

- White blond, ash/warm ash blond, dark ash blond

- Ash brown, dark brown (taupe tone)

- Brown with auburn cast
- Blue-gray or pearl white

EYES:

- Blue (with white webbing in iris, a cloudy look)
- Green (with white webbing in iris, a cloudy look)
- Soft gray-blue, soft gray-green
- Bright clear blue, pale clear aqua (eyes change from blue to green, depending on clothes)
- Hazel (cloudy brown smudge with blue or green)
- Pale gray
- Soft rose brown or grayed brown

JEWELRY:

- Silver tone is best

AUTUMN colors are likened to typical colors we see in the fall: salmon pink, light peach, terra-cotta, jade, rust, olive, gold, pumpkin, and mahogany.

You will look best in AUTUMN (warm) colors if:

SKIN:

- Ivory or ivory with freckles (usually a redhead)
- Peach or peach with freckles (usually golden blond or brown)
- Golden beige, dark beige (coppery), or golden brown

HAIR:

- Red or auburn
- Coppery brown
- Golden honey blond or golden brown (dark honey)
- Dirty or strawberry blond
- Charcoal brown or black

- Golden gray or oyster white

EYES:

- Dark brown , golden brown

- Amber, hazel, golden brown, green gold

- Green with brown or gold flecks, clear green, or olive green

- Steel blue, teal blue, or bright turquoise

JEWELRY:

- Gold tone is best

After determining which season's palette you believe most flatters you, you'll find that shopping for clothes gets much easier. This is mostly because it eliminates a lot of temptations such as sale price, brand name, or whose style you simply like. Knowing what colors to look for and what ones to avoid gives you more confidence to say, "No, thank you; I think I'll pass!"

Another great benefit is that you'll save money. How? It's simple. When you have a wardrobe of articles in the same color season, making new outfits from existing ones is a lot less complicated. Mixing and matching is effortless, so you get more outfits from the same number of pieces. Plus, finding good deals can turn into quick purchases because you don't have to think about whether you might have something at home to wear with the particular top. When it's a fabric in the right family, you probably have a myriad of options.

Color affects people differently. Wear colors that make YOU feel great and look fresh and that make your skin glow and you'll look and feel like the leader of the pack. Sprinkle in a little personality and a few accessories to pull it all together and voila! You've got a "knockout" total package, no matter how you look at it. So don't settle for the view from the back . . . It never changes. Get out there and lead the way!

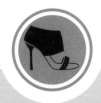

STEP UP TO ACTION:

A Rainbow of Rave Reviews

Do I lean more toward wearing warm or cool colors? Refer to the color chart in the photo section if you still need clarification.

When I wear neutrals (black, gray, brown, cream, white, and true red), what one color do I love to use for an accent?

What season best represents the color family I should incorporate most in my wardrobe?

What one color can I recall definitely being "NOT so good" on me?

How can I use the meaning of color to my advantage (wardrobe, home décor, office, etc.)?

Chapter 6

GLAMOUR AND GLITZ: DO YOU NEED A CHECKUP FROM THE NECK UP?

I really love this topic because it's the quickest, easiest fix around! A new tube of lipstick can be the best "outfit accessory," a new hairstyle or color can give the illusion of looking ten pounds lighter, and proper eye makeup application truly allows them to be the window to the soul. To suit the average woman's lifestyle needs, she should have about three various glamour looks in her repertoire of options for taking her color cosmetics adventure from naked to knockout. (Even if you are a minimalist, a little bit of color is recommended. Refer to my "dash out the door" approach to keep things subtle.) If you are a working woman or simply someone who prefers the magical style of sophisticated transformation daily, then the tips in this chapter will be of great interest to you. For that special-occasion makeup that goes from polished to pizzazz, here are a few extra tips: in general, add an extra coat of mascara (or fake eyelashes!), lip liner and gloss are a must, add a crystalline highlighter with a bit of shimmer on the brow bone of the eye and a dot in the inside corner nearest your nose, define those brows, and buff on a bit of bronzer for a shimmer finish.

Dressing from the neck up should be given as much attention as dressing from the neck down. Thank goodness we have products that diminish fine lines, tighten pores, hide discolorations, and fill in lines, plus colors from every shade of the rainbow to paint on lots of different places. While you don't need to be an artist to have a great makeup application, it does help to know some tips and tricks. This encompasses your skin care regime, foundation fundamentals, hairstyle and condition, lip color, eye color application, having brows that "wow," and beautiful bronzers—but remember that it all starts with keeping your skin in the best shape possible so that it will last you a lifetime.

Facing up to Skin Care

While good makeup application includes using the right colors as well as the right tools (brushes, sponges, and the like) and techniques, it actually starts with well-cared-for skin. There are four basic skin types: dry, normal, combination or "T" zone (more oily on forehead, nose, and chin area), and oily. Since human skin generates new skin cells every three to four days, it's important to slough off the older dead ones at least twice a week. And while we're touching on the topic of old skin cells, it helps to understand that your skin is likely to change over the years thanks to the effects of the natural aging process, diet, and hormones. So will your hair. Certain medications, menopause, and pregnancy all additionally affect the look and feel of skin and hair.

Knowing your skin type is important for choosing the most appropriate skin care product line, but like anything else, "follow the money." What someone recommends might be driven more by profits than your best interest. Finding a quality skin care regime is not hard or costly and at its most basic should include a cleanser and moisturizer with sunscreen for daily use. Additional preferred products include eye creams, toners, exfoliators/masks for weekly use, body scrubs to diminish dead skin cells, and nighttime products that replenish skin's lost nutrients and vitamins and add elasticity. Use products with peptides (wrinkle-fighting proteins that are key to collagen synthesis and enhance the performance of antioxidants). Many natural ingredient extracts are being used for their restoring, hydrating, replenishing, and stabilizing benefits. Pay attention to pomegranate, acai berry, chestnut seed, aloe, sunflower seed, kakadu plum, and cucumber, to name a few powerful ones.

Some people rave about great results they get with at-home natural concoctions for skin and hair, using cucumber, aloe, and pumpkin masks, vinegar, egg yolk washes for hair, oatmeal and sea salt combos

for skin . . . and the list goes on. There are many Web sites that list recipes and have pictures and testimonies; I've had great results creating
my own, especially with my two girls. It's fun and healthy to be organic.
The challenge in choosing to avoid products with certain chemicals (the
"all-natural" approach, for instance) is that the shortened life span of the
items you buy can be equally as detrimental as those with preservatives.
This is a personal choice you have to make based on the best products
for you and your skin type, lifestyle, and, of course, preference. And as
your skin changes over the years, it's likely the products you'll need will,
too. Spending a lot of money on products that don't work is a frustration
we all share. That's why a "try before you buy" approach is so helpful. Try
some and see what works for you, but don't be fooled by thinking that if
a product costs more, it must be better. It's simply a myth and a busted
one at that!

And last but not least, some advice you've probably heard a million
times but warrants repeating:

**Two tried-and-true tips for great skin are
(1) always wear sunscreen and (2) drink more water!**

FOUNDATIONS

A makeup foundation is both the final step in quality skin care and the
first step in providing a neutral canvas for color. Again, it starts with
good skin care, and then you add the extras. It's like baking a cake. You
start with the essential ingredients (flour, sugar, oil, eggs), and then you
add the extras. Finally, you add the icing . . . the glamour makeup!

One thing women invariably ask me for assistance with is how to get
the perfect foundation match for a truly flawless finish. They most often
do not want to look or feel like they have a lot of makeup on, which is a
good thing. Choosing the right foundation begins with understanding
your skin type (dry, normal, combo, or oily) and knowing what you want
your foundation to do. From there, we decide what color and formula
are best for you. Sheer liquids can provide a lighter coverage, which is

great if you're a minimalist. Others prefer a creamier, fuller coverage to hide flaws and provide a more even finish that covers any discolorations their skin may have. When using a cream or liquid foundation, the most important step is the tool: foundation applied with a custom foundation brush will give you a truly flawless finish, is more sanitary, and makes blending a cinch. You really must try it if you don't already use one. There are brands in every type under the sun to choose from. I recommend finding someone you can work with to ensure that you are getting a perfect match and who allows you to experience different formulas. To achieve a matte finish, simply apply a mineral powder formula, either alone or over a liquid, to "set" the look.

Some folks wonder about using additional products to get the desired end result with their foundation. For example, whether to use a concealer depends on what you're trying to accomplish; if you have specific areas and imperfections that need more coverage, a concealer might be a good idea. Another product to try is a facial highlighting pen to brighten any darker areas. Mary Kay Cosmetics has an awesome one, and many of the makeup artists at the CMA Awards used it on their celebrity makeovers. There should be a balance of both highlighting and concealing areas on your face. Under-eye circles seem to be the number one area most women want to brighten. A good eye cream will contain vitamin K and antioxidants and do more than just moisturize. Read the labels; products with those ingredients will address the real issue and keep your peepers from looking like creepers. Then double up by using a concealer under your foundation and a highlighting pen in a slightly lighter color than your naked skin and dab it in the inner corner of your nose/eye area. It works wonders to brighten up tired, dark, and droopy eyes.

HAIR

If you haven't received a compliment on your hair in the past six months, then it's time for a new "do." But what kind of "do" should you do? If you don't know after looking through endless magazines, you can hopefully trust the judgment of your respected hairdresser. When looking for the right stylist for you, consider these criteria: Do your personalities mesh? Is he or she consistent and timely? Does he or she participate in continuing-education classes? Does he or she do a good job AND teach you care and maintenance on your hair? Does he or she make new recommendations for seasonal updates? Is the salon clean, well kept, and organized? Is there a sense of rapport among the staff? If you are going to spend an hour a month with him or her, you want to make sure it's a pleasant experience, meaning that you are in the hands of a skilled technician and you get service worth remembering . . . and passing on. Most salons will want this kind of positive response from their clients as well since they know that their biggest marketing tool is word of mouth!

According to a local hair and spa salon, the need to shampoo daily is a myth. "It's simply not necessary," says Brenda Wittman, owner of Surface Colorspa in downtown Mount Dora, Florida. In this case, **less can be more**, and this seems to be a trend in much of the fashion industry. Since about 2009, the philosophy for hair, makeup, and accessories is that less is more; simple and elegant can go hand in hand. And since you lose so much of your hair, anyway, overprocessing can turn into a detriment rather than a benefit. An average head loses 80–100 hairs per day, and the life cycle of hair takes seven years to complete. That means that without even trying, you'll have a new head of hair and possibly a new "do" every seven years. Most of us can't or won't wait that long! So, ladies, check your mane. Are you losing it? If so, that's a normal and healthy sign. If you're not losing some hair, it could be a sign of a health issue that has sent your hair growth into the resting stage. This is very common during pregnancy, which is why you lose so much of it *after* the baby comes.

By the time you reach fifty percent gray, it's time to go one to two shades lighter. "It's nature's way of telling us to 'lighten up,'" Wittman says. Gray tends to have a little less moisture, so an extra or new conditioner may be in order. Changing up your product use can produce positive results so that your hair doesn't build up resistance. A good hair designer can assess your specific needs and recommend formulas best suited for you.

Hairstyles present another challenge. For some, it's a daily one, and yet others are fine with a six-week cycle at their favorite salon. So how do you choose one that fits YOU?

Start by knowing what your face shape really is. I know that sounds silly; after all, you've been living with it all your life, right? But we can easily confuse our actual face shape with the shape that shows based on our current hairstyle. Next time you're in front of the mirror, hold your hair back with a headband and see what your face shape really is. After determining that, you can utilize a style (and glamour makeup!) to create balance and a harmonized look.

Bangs or no bangs? If you have a diamond, rectangle, or classic oval face, then they work great. If you have a square, circle, or heart-shaped face, they're not so good. According to Wittman, the goal of a good cut is to flatter your face shape by creating an ideal oval. Bangs create a bold horizontal line right across your forehead, so if that isn't your goal, you might want to try a side part. The modern shag is an example of a hairstyle that will compliment most all face shapes.

Here are some simple guidelines:

Circle or full face: Lightly layered, sweeps below the ear

Heart shaped: Side part, keep hair away from the face; if it's long enough, try a flip at the shoulder

Square: Layers toward the face will help soften a strong jawline

Diamond: Needs bangs, similar to the heart shape

Rectangle: Needs bangs and wispiness; curls can be good

With oodles of opportunity for extensions to add hair fullness or length, straight irons to flatten frizzy hair, spiral curling irons for creating major curls, product to hold it all together, and retailers providing every style of "hair pretty" you can imagine, there's no reason why a new "do" can't be in store for you. Jazz up your appearance with a surprise element. It's youthful and a great way to get you out of the same-old, same-old doldrums. One of the most common challenges I hear from my clients is "I'm in a rut doing the same thing every day." Here's a perfect way to break out: add a flower or classy crystal on a bobby pin to your flowing (or spiky) mane and smile! It works wonders at any age.

ADD THE ICING . . .
AND SPRINKLES, PLEASE

The other way to create an instant update is with your glamour colors. Since lipstick and mascara are the two most universally sold cosmetics, I will address the lip color issue. Being a businesswoman myself, I cannot imagine why a woman wouldn't be wearing any lipstick, but it happens. If that's you, here's an interesting bit of not-so-trivial trivia that might inspire you to change:

Women who wear lipstick earn approximately eighty percent more money than those who do not.

Finding the right shade for you is the trick. You can refer to the section on color and determine whether you look better in warm or cool tones and start there. Assuming you are a "cool" tone, you'll stick with pinks, berries, and reds with blue undertones. There is a fine line of overlap between the shades of pink, and to say you cannot wear "pink" is a disservice to yourself. For a neutral pink tone, you'll want colors that are more mild, muted, and blended with a soft brown/beige. A coral liner coupled with a pink lipstick will create a version of peach or tawny pink and is appropriate for those with warmer undertones.

Generally speaking, softer pastels look better on fair skin or someone younger than thirty-five. Why? Because as we mature, our skin not only loses elasticity but also begins to lose its color (along with a lot of other things that begin to sag, droop, and creak, oh my!). If you're over forty, my best advice with lip color is (1) never leave home without it; (2) use liner to fill in and define the entire lip area; (3) occasionally use a lip exfoliator so that they stay looking plump, moist, and rid of dry flakes; and (4) apply a color that is brighter rather than darker. A shade such as raspberry, fuchsia, citrus, or plum is better than a pale mauve or deep fig, raisin, or bronze. Because color is so personal, you really do need to customize your look by trying the colors out and not guessing. Lipstick colors often change once they are applied and have combined with your natural coloring. We especially see this in women whose lips naturally have very bright red or blue undertones. You will also want to consider the season of the year for optimum color choices. You don't want to still be wearing the same lip color in the summer that you were wearing back during the holidays.

Did you know that you can tell someone's personality by the shape of her lipstick? It's true . . . and when you register on my Web site, simply click on the link for the downloadable version of "THE LIPSTICK PERSONALITY" and give it a try. I would love your feedback to see how accurate my "test" is. It's a great tool for office women to compare and girlfriends to share. Have fun and you're welcome!

EYES AND BROWS

Having brows that say "WOW" doesn't mean you have to get tweezed, watery eyed, and red skinned. Almost no one has a perfectly symmetrical face, but learning how and where to apply color on your face to create balance is a good thing, and that includes your brows. They should have their highest arch on approximately the outer one-third of the eye and then taper down from there. Take a pencil and extend it diagonally from the outer edge of your nostril to the outer corner of your eyeball. The place where that diagonal line reaches your brow is where the brow should end. This helps define whether you pluck the strays that extend too far or whether you may need to add a little eyebrow pencil to fill in and extend as necessary. If you're filling in, select a color closest to your natural brow coloring; here it's best to opt for a shade lighter so as to appear more natural. If you do not have any brows at all (this happens with many older women or those enduring cancer treatment), this is a technique you will want to master. Brow powder is best applied with a sharp, firm brush.

It's my goal to have all my clients say, "EYE can do that!" Applying eye makeup with finesse really does take practice, and over the years I've become quite a master. The number one request I hear from my clients is "Teach me how to do my eyes." Apparently this is number one for women around the world as well, based on what I've read over the years. The magazines are loaded with visuals, how-to's, pictures, recommended products, and trendy colors.

My advice? Have a minimum of six colors, three to form an everyday natural palette and three more for a classic to dramatic look. Examples of natural colors can be a flesh tone in cream or taupe for the base, a darker medium brown to contour in the crease, and a softer vanilla to highlight the brow bone area. For drama or glam, the smoky eye is always in; for that kind of look, most all eye and skin tone colors can use the same taupe base color (go more golden for a "warm" effect, and go more soft pale pink for a "cool" effect, as you just learned in the previous chapter). Your other two options should have depth; think smoky plum, smoky silver-black, or bold navy for your contour color and another midtone for blending.

And don't forget the *"EYE gotta have it" must have item of the year*: a shimmery white eye color! Use this for blending, highlighting the brow bone, softening colors that might be too dark, AND the biggest trick of all . . . to "dot" the inner corner of the eye closest to your nose to lighten up those dark areas. It's THE WAY to create an instant wake-up with your peepers. Try it. It's so simple . . . BLEND, BLEND, BLEND! Use a sponge-tipped applicator to avoid having the powder "flick" everywhere; use a blending brush for the finish.

Last but not least, the mascara. Start with the eyelash curler; if you don't have one, get one! Always use it before applying mascara rather than after so as to avoid breaking any lashes. Open the curler and place the upper eyelashes into the mouth of the curler. Squeeze and hold steady for a slow count of five and then release. Next, swipe the mascara wand once or twice on the side of the tube to remove any clumps from the wand. Place the wand at the middle of your eyelid and hold still while rolling the wand up and outward. This helps keep you from poking yourself and messing up the entire eye look and having to start over. Move the wand to the inner part of the eyelash area and repeat. Finish by accenting the outer third of the eyelashes and really defining them with the boldest amount of product. Pull those outer lashes up and away from the outer corner to create more glam and open up the eye area. A light dusting on the bottom lashes is equally as important. Voila! You now have movie star allure without the hassle of falsies. Go on . . . love your lashes.

BRONZERS

We all want a golden glow. While it is true that the vitamin D you get from natural sunlight is really healthy, the damaging effects of the sun's UV rays may get you thinking twice about alternative methods for a safe golden glow. There are options for giving your face and your body a luminous and sun-kissed complexion in a safe and fairly inexpensive way besides the tanning bed. Self-tanning products have come a long, long way since their invention a few decades ago, so don't be afraid to give one a try.

Before applying it, though, be sure to exfoliate the areas you are targeting. This sloughs off dead or dry skin cells and allows the tanning lotion to blend into your pores more easily; it also helps avoid any color streaks. You can use a buffing cream for extra smoothness. When you apply a self-tanning lotion, you must allow it to dry fully before getting dressed so that the product doesn't discolor your clothing.

The results of a tanning lotion can last about a week. For a deep, blended tan, apply at night, the following morning, and again that night. And of course, depending on the shade you want to achieve, more applications may be necessary. If "stink, stank, and stunk" are some keywords that you associate with using these products, then I've got good news: they have gotten much better smelling! But do a sniff test for yourself BEFORE purchasing and find out about a return policy in case you have any allergy issues or are generally unhappy with the results. If you love the smell of a piña colada and want to imagine yourself bathing on the beaches of the Bahamas, you're in luck . . . Most have adopted a tropical scent.

According to leading dermatologists, lotions that change the color of skin pigmentation are far safer than tanning beds.

Standing and indulging in a spray tan method is another option. Most tanning salons offer this, and it proves to be a real time saver. The process generally takes about ten to fifteen minutes; you actually stand while being physically sprayed with a dye that turns your skin instantly bronze. This method, though also temporary, could be a great answer for special-occasion needs.

Yet another way to achieve a safe (but temporary) bronze complexion is to simply purchase facial cosmetics, such as a mineral powder bronzer in a loose or pressed formula. When applying bronzer to the facial area, think of the most common places that actual sunlight would hit: your cheeks, nose, and forehead. With a fluffy brush, blend the bronzer across these areas, and don't forget to include the décolleté, shoulders, or back if you have a strapless top or tank on.

I love working with a bronzer because of its multiple uses. Try it as an eye color since it usually comes mixed with various light and dark bronze pigments. Some are matte, and some are shimmery; best results happen when you blend both. It's usually a good product for most skin types and colors, though not everyone looks good in a bronzy undertone. Skin that is too sallow or has yellow undertones may not be able to pull off this look. Be wary of using a copper lip color when you also have facial bronzer; the results are often too metallic. While some bronzers are too ruddy, others can be too orange or golden. Finding the right hue for you might take some practice, but it'll be worth it.

Putting it all together will work whether your style best represents a "No-Fuss Fannie" approach, a "Classic Carrie," or a "Glamorous Gloria" one. Regardless of your general preferences, you can achieve a basic look by making a bronzer your cosmetic BFF. How? By making it the basis of your five-minute "dash-out-the-door" look:

Keep bronzer, mascara, eye pencil, and lip color in your cosmetic bag so you can dash out the door, LOOK IN THE REARVIEW MIRROR, AND LIKE WHAT YOU SEE!

Like jewelry, makeup is also an accessory . . . but again, I refer to it as a necessary accessory! Some women have convictions not to wear any; some resist, thinking that the "natural" way is the only way to truly be empowered; and others overuse it, unable to leave the house without a two-hour daily ritual. Somewhere in the middle works best for me. "Harmony" is the word that comes to mind. When your inner beauty matches your outer beauty, you are most empowered to fulfill whatever your life's purpose is, and those around you will believe it, too. The more our inner strength is reinforced by our outer image, the more effective and successful we can be.

"For attractive lips, speak words of kindness. For lovely eyes, seek out the good in people. For a slim figure, share your food with the hungry. For beautiful hair, let a child run his or her fingers through it once a day. For poise, walk with the knowledge that you never walk alone. People, even more than things, have to be restored, renewed, revived, reclaimed, and redeemed; never throw out anyone. Remember, if you ever need a helping hand, you will find one at the end of each of your arms. As you grow older, you will discover that you have two hands; one for helping yourself, and the other for helping others."

—Attributed to Sam Levenson and
often quoted by Audrey Hepburn

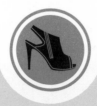

STEP UP TO ACTION:

Tips and Tricks for Must-Have Makeup

A checkup from the neck up can help you determine your skin type (dry, oily, combo, or normal). Ask yourself, "Am I getting optimum results from the regime I'm currently using?"

Using cosmetics is one way to bring out your best. Decide what your best feature is (eyes, brows, hair, cheekbones, flawless skin tone, lips) and work on enhancing it.

Do I need to wash my brushes or replace them?

Download the complimentary lipstick personality chart from my Web site (www.NakedtoKnockout.com) and see whether the shape of your tube matches your personality.

PURCHASE AT LEAST ONE NEW LIPSTICK COLOR
FOR EACH SEASON.

Chapter 7

DRESS TO IMPRESS,
FOR LESS, AND FOR SUCCESS

Does the way you dress communicate success? Does it at least send the message you intended it to?

You might say it doesn't matter to your friends or neighbors, but at the very least, you should agree that it does matter when it comes to your career prospects. As I'm writing this, the stock market's volatility continues, and unemployment has been hanging around nine percent for many months. If you have a job, this chapter could help you improve your options for keeping it . . . and if you are looking for one, this chapter is definitely for you. If you want to recession proof your image, start here. The ideas I am presenting will also be cost-effective for you in the long run.

Job seekers know that by the time they get to the interview, their potential new employer has found out many things about them based on their résumé and other background checks. Getting to a live interview means their general appearance, manners, body language, and communication skills are going to be assessed to see whether they're the right "fit" for the position. It's not unusual for a qualified person not to get the job because he or she lacks the image necessary. This is so important to grasp. Consider these statistics:

7% of success depends on WHAT you say—Content
38% of success depends on HOW you say it—Tonality
45% of success depends on WHAT you LOOK like—Physiology

From these numbers, I urge you to give some real attention to your appearance during job interviews and when networking for business growth. As a professional in any field, it adds credibility to look like one. It matters! This will also help you know where to focus most of your time and attention in preparing for the perfect presentation or appointment. In this chapter I will define some dressing styles, discuss appropriate attire for business, and cover a few basic etiquette points.

PROPER PREPARATION PREVENTS POOR PERFORMANCE

Granted, the information here is basic since many other factors need to be considered, such as whether the job is in government, upper-level industry, sales, corporate, etc. You will have a better chance for a better job at a higher salary when you learn how to use clothing as a business tool. If you are like many entrepreneurs and are using YouTube as a marketing tool, you want to be sure that what you're wearing is visually appealing on camera—it might just keep the viewer from pushing the "stop" button after the first ten seconds. And if you are a speaker, the impression you make determines almost instantly whether you'll engage your audience or be dismissed. You can be sure that an interviewer can spot the difference between a $100 suit and a $1,000 one. While a suit valued at $100 may be fine to wear *on the job*, the other will be a good investment for helping you *get the job*. Use the following checklist to help make a great impression at your next big appointment, whether you are a guy or a gal.

- *Suit yourself:* Ninety-five percent of the time, you can't go wrong wearing a suit. Everyone should own at least one good one. (I am not suggesting you need a $1,000 suit to make a great impression or even interview in for that matter. The price doesn't necessarily matter; the quality does.)
- Convey confidence by looking right eye to right eye.
- Make sure your bangs do not hang in or hide your face. Most people will not trust you if they cannot see your eyes, so to avoid being thought of as a shady character, get a new hairdo or simply wear it up.

- Bring a clean notebook portfolio to take notes in, with a pen that preferably costs more than one dollar and does not have the end chewed off.

- Extend your hand for the handshake first upon entering and remember to call the interviewer by name.

- Although the appointment is about you, make it your job to find out something about the other person. Be prepared with two key questions, such as "How long have you worked here?" and "What do you like best about it?"

- Shoes should be free of any scuffs and in good repair.

- Teeth and nails are very visible, so keep them clean. Enough said.

A suit in stretch wool fabric is seasonless and doesn't easily wrinkle. A dark charcoal mini-pinstripe is good on almost all body shapes because it adds height and you can pair it with a variety of shells. Choose one with a pencil skirt; add a solid-color button-front blouse or a scoop-neck shell in a flattering color. Make sure everything is ironed and the buttons do not pull, and keep jewelry simple. Diamond studs or classic pearl earrings are best. This is not the time for anything that jingles, is clanky, or causes you to fidget. The shoes must be a classic closed-toe pump in average heel; no stilettos or flats. Finish the look with nude hose and very light or preferably no perfume. If you opt for a pantsuit, make sure that the pockets do not poke and gather unnecessarily and that the hem is hanging perfectly for the size heel you wear. Be sure the jacket really "fits." This is the one piece that makes or breaks the outfit, and it must flatter you.

Many other dressing-for-success tips can be found in the book *Dress for Success*, written by the father of the subject, John T. Molloy. I have utilized his principles and statistics (based on years of studies he performed) and then tweaked them to relate to modern-day acceptance. While we are a much more relaxed society than we were back in the eighties, many of his principles still ring true. Dress-down Fridays have become the norm in most banks and schools, including universities.

What hasn't changed is the message that gets conveyed when you miss the mark for making a great first impression. It can absolutely cost you in terms of missed opportunities—for hire, for promotion, for networking, and more. If you want to land an important deal or be taken more seriously, take note and always dress "up" a level. Read on for tips on how to do this and still be comfortable in your own skin. We'll actually start with wardrobe economics—how to successfully dress for success for less. Trust me!

WARDROBE ECONOMICS

A dress-for-less mentality is something I have practiced for a long time. I married the man who owned jeans and T-shirts (with one pocket on the front and words only on the back) as his wardrobe staple and who thought *all* department stores were *all* overpriced, *all* the time, and that the only reasonable place to shop was Wal-Mart. We've come a long way in twenty years. To say I was slightly different is, ahem, being kind.

It's hard to resist the bargain temptations, but if you're like most of us, you've had your fair share of bargain-buying boo-boos . . . those things that seemed like such a great deal at the time, only to fall apart after one wearing or else they don't go with anything, anytime, anywhere. Disciplining ourselves not to give in to such temptations can actually save money over time.

You can easily adopt the principle of "buy the best quality you can for the best price you can afford." It was easy to prove that ten discount-store golf shirts needed to be replaced before ten Ralph Lauren ones did. I am not saying shopping at the big-box discounters is a waste. To the contrary . . . just know the main value you're investing in and the return you're hoping to get. I suspect this philosophy is resonating with you right now. A poorly made garment will fade more quickly, will not last through twenty washes (which is wearing the item less than two times a month for one year!), and will probably need to be altered or repaired after just a few wearings. These are some of the reasons why I love shopping at Stein Mart. It's a perfect blend, in my opinion, of quality, quantity, and affordable pricing. Those benefits, along with the "experience" you get walking into Stein Mart versus other discount stores, are why I will always travel the extra miles to get there. It's a worthwhile treat.

The other consideration I find when comparing best investment buys is to look at national chains versus local boutiques. Believe me, I shop at them all, and guess what? I have found some incredible wardrobe investments, steals, one-of-a-kinds, and made-just-for-me pieces at small, quaint boutiques. Apart from the fact that I love frequenting these places in the cities I travel, I have also found that their designers have an amazing flair for sizing, especially for those with "unique shapes." Simply put, if you're repeatedly frustrated by the way pants from the chain stores fit, for example, then break out of your comfort zone and try a local boutique. You might be pleasantly surprised.

Furthermore, when you shop local, you are doing a major favor to your economy by boosting it! I love frequenting local shops in my area and haveenjoyed developing relationships with many different kinds of local boutique owners and enjoy sending clients their way. And they reciprocate: because they know your style, don't be surprised if you get a call offering to set aside some really great piece that just arrived so you can get the first shot at it! You might pay more up front, but the service, wearability, uniqueness, and longevity of the garment will often equal or be less than other pieces purchased through retail department stores.

Retail chains offer their own list of benefits, from their wide assortment of brands and size options to online shopping, overnight delivery, the convenience of "total look" shopping (shoes, bags, accessories, hose, undergarments, and so on), and even some major sales (one of their most endearing qualities!). Sign up for frequent VIP customer programs to receive the biggest bang for your buck. Some of them also offer personal shopping assistance. The downside? Because they deal in such quantities, you're likely at some point to run into someone else in the same outfit. And beware of their strategic devices to lure you into spending more than you need to just to take advantage of the "special." That said, I confess that Chico's and Cache are two of my favorites. They do a great job of providing quality, current, and on-trend styles that will help you make a style statement, and they offer specials that keep their pricing generally affordable.

In developing a style all your own, you have probably developed a "shopping style" all your own, too. Change it up; variety is the spice of life. Being too predictable is just plain boring. And you, my dear, should be anything but boring!

Now, let's get busy.

THE BARE ESSENTIALS

Having undergarments that fit you and are comfortable may seem like an impossibility. Necessary indeed and since we should wear them daily, it's a great idea to find a bra that is your perfect fit. My friend Ali Cudby is a FAB foundation expert, and she can help you with this intimate issue. (Please refer to the resource guide to contact her.) My opinion is limited and personal: know when to give your girls a lift and when to let the ta-tas breathe. Between Victoria's Secret, Spanx, L'eggs, Fredericks of Hollywood, and Maidenform, they've got you covered. Having hose, panties, bras, and slips that smooth or hide any excess, provide protection, and deliver a dynamic foundation is one way to start your daily dressing regime with a style all your own. Don't leave home without it!

FASHION VERSUS STYLE

Is there really such a thing as a timeless fashion style?

We hear the phrase all the time, but it's not accurate. Fashion relates to more trendy "come-and-go" clothing designs, whereas style is about you—how you use clothing to represent your personality. More than just a matter of taste, style also means knowing how to build a versatile wardrobe by buying quality rather than quantity, purchasing items that work well with your existing wardrobe (or the new one you are building!), and investing in "timeless" pieces, meaning they can be worn for seasons to come. Such pieces become very affordable on a cost-per-wear basis.

Being predictable in your clothing and opting for only neutrals (beige, denim, white or cream, black, gray, and brown) can get boring (or at least "basic"). A more conservative dresser will have a wardrobe full of these pieces and will benefit greatly from the next chapter on how to accessorize. In fact, most women describe their style to me by including that word: boring. That isn't any way to express your best self to the world and let your inner beauty shine. Knowing how to go from a "boring/naked" canvas to creating a "knockout" one is what this book is all about. We could learn our lessons on this category from the stars alone and follow one popular thought: "I base most of my fashion sense on what doesn't itch" (Gilda Radner). While we laugh, there are a lot of people following that advice.

There are generally two main categories of style: **classic/conservative** and **dramatic/high impact**. Your personal style is going to fall mostly into one camp or the other, with a variety of subcategories in each one that might better describe you. Many people who have studied the history of fashion may have far differing viewpoints from mine; all I am trying to do is provide a basic platform for the average woman to build her wardrobe on. With that said, let's look at the variations within the two categories.

CLASSIC/CONSERVATIVE

The classic clothing personality is a sign of grace and tasteful style. Clean, straight lines dominate your closet. You prefer to keep your outfit simple and highlight your personality, and you have a tendency to match your clothes. You avoid loud, faddish trends.

Your celebrity style twins: Chanel, Jackie O, Katie Holmes (classic and sporty), Brooke Shields, Lauren Conrad (classic and trendy), and Angelina Jolie (classic and minimalist).

Women who dress like this tend to be a bit on the safe side. To extend your comfort zone, try adding a scarf, a bold pop of color to your neutrals, or a high-impact piece of jewelry. Also, try stretching your style by selecting your essentials in a different color than a neutral; for example, if you're into ballet flats, see whether you can try a new pair with a bow or some gold hardware. Opt for a colorful shell to pop against that cream-colored suit.

DRAMATIC/HIGH IMPACT

So vogue. A dramatic clothing personality commands attention and can both intimidate and intrigue. This preference tends to avoid frilly accessories. You like creating a strong and distinctive fashion statement. And this is a reflection of your bold personality. Making a high impact is important to you, and your confidence is expressed with your clothing. You're into the latest fashion trends but like showing off some authority in the way you dress. You might even embrace an eclectic approach with your casual and sporty choices. For evening, you're sure to shine as any diva should in sequins, glitter, and diamonds. You tend to choose clothes with angular necklines, shapes, and edges, such as jackets with shoulder pads, and you're into diagonal abstract prints.

Your celebrity style twins: Fran Drescher, Monica Bellucci, Megan Fox, Anne Hathaway, Dita von Teese, and the ultimate, Lady Gaga.

Another "branch" from this style is the socialite who loves to dress a bit glamorous but polished and likes to convey a sense of status; she probably carries a couture bag from Dolce and Gabbana, Big Buddha, or Chanel. Enhancing your style will include pieces such as strong Art Deco jewelry, cuffs, gemstones, and tops with angular or padded shoulders. The warning for you is not to overdo it. Pay careful attention to your occasion and how others will be dressed. Playing down your look is one way to soften your edge. Your fashion forwardness can be intimidating to both men and women, and you don't want to risk being mistaken. Think "classic" and you'll probably be fine.

Whether you opt for classic/conservative or dramatic/high impact, there are other styles that you can reference when creating a style all your own. **French fashion** is one of the chicest looks you can achieve.

En vogue fashion is highly influenced by the French, who are considered to be the sole founders and true pioneers of style. It's classy but a bit sassy.

It's not difficult to look like you stepped out of a Paris café. Chic and sleek are what I associate with French womenswear. You may get inspired to implement the "less is more" philosophy used by French women for several decades. From Chanel to Givenchy, they all share the same vision: TIMELESS, SOPHISTICATED, AND FEMININE. If that is a style you are comfortable in, you'll shop for a couture-ish fur or leather jacket, almost always be in a blazer of some sort, and have very tailored clothing. You can easily notice French women's simplicity in their style, and yet they have a discreet sexiness that can make any man fall off his feet. What really sets French women apart from the rest is their sense of style, which is not the same thing as wearing the hottest trends. It's been said that fashion can be bought but style one must possess.

Vintage wear is unique because it helps us connect a part of the past with an update of today. I like vintage styles because they are economical and great conversation starters. You can often create a wow factor because of the unique tailoring, details, fabrics, or overall style. Today's fashion has been recycled from all different eras: dramatic Art Deco twenties and thirties, tailored forties and fifties, flowing hippie sixties and seventies, and a rock-urban period in the eighties, so really, there's something for everyone! Note that "vintage" doesn't mean "the reeeally old kind of Victorian styles." Vintage, well, it doesn't really go out of style, so plunge into the past and discover how vintage handbags, T-shirts, dresses, and sweaters can take your look to another level.

Another option is **Bohemian**. It's a casual mix of hippie, ethnic, gypsy, and vintage elements and really easy to create. Plus, it's comfortable. Kate Moss and Mary Kate Olsen are the celebs who pull off this style with flair. How do they do it? Snoop around; their Boho shopping secrets are not so secret anymore, thanks to the Internet. Many women try to pull this off but often end up looking like street beggars, with too many heavy pieces that drag down instead of lifting up the look. A platform shoe with a Boho scarf, cute jeggings, and a gypsy tunic is enough.

Heaps of accessories are not needed. Finding your own niche to connect classic with Boho is essential. Boho fashion is considered a state of mind rather than "just a fashion trend that will fade in time."

Once you have defined your own style, you can begin dressing for success in a way that helps you feel confident and sexy in your own skin. Fashion will clearly come and go . . . but a woman with style remains. Eve wore fig leaves; a lot has changed since then. Knowing how to find your style of clothing and where to find it can be simplified when you use the resource guide at the back of this book. With the benefits of online shopping, you can Google almost any topic and style of dress and find many retailers. Check on their return policy. One I love is Zappos, not only because of free shipping and free returns, great style options, variety of sizes almost always available, and great customer service but also because I love their story and align with Tony Hsieh's mission. Check them out if you haven't already at www.zappos.com.

Many online retailers are driven to accommodate at-home shoppers looking for value and service. I do shop online, but that convenience will never replace the experience for me of hunting for that great find. Most men understand "the hunt." For me, shopping is no different . . . and it's a lot more exciting and rewarding than sitting in a tree stand with a shotgun. I should know. I tried wearing a mink in the woods, my rhinestones while hiking, and stilettos to Disney. It's just not the same thrill.

ETIQUETTE

The first impression you make includes your smile and handshake. Did you know that forty percent of all adults have social anxiety and that seventy-five percent experience some anxiety at a party with strangers? Boost your confidence by extending the proper handshake and salutation when meeting others for the first time. A correct shake includes fingers together with your thumb up to connect with the other in a comfortable grasp. Many women make the mistake of a finger-tip approach that leaves others with a limp, wimpy sense of who you are. Be firm and confident, but don't be a bone crusher! This is simply overkill for men and women. It used to be seen more as a power move, but it really is a matter of respect. I will respect you more for sure when you don't grip so tightly that my rings dig into my flesh, thank you!

Here are some other helpful tips to use when greeting others and for making introductions:

- Say the name of the person you want to give the greatest honor to first.

- A customer's name is spoken before that of anyone in your organization, including the CEO.

- Professionally, age and gender play no part in whose name is spoken first.

- The name of an elected official or a member of the clergy is spoken first regardless of gender.

- Only mention each person's name once. Example: Don't say, "Betty Smith, this is Ted Jenkins. Ted Jenkins, this is Betty Smith." The correct phrase to use is: "Betty Smith, I'd like to introduce you to Ted Jenkins."

- Always add a little about each person so they can begin a conversation if you step away.

- Customers and clients should be referred to by their honorific or title until they ask you to call them by their first name.

- The proper honorific for all women at work is "Ms." unless they request otherwise.

The above principles work well with phone etiquette, too. Remember those statistics from the beginning of the chapter? Thirty-eight percent of success is in how you say it, and this is extremely important when you are on the phone because other people do not have the benefit of seeing what you look like. They can, however, hear a smile!

WHEN YOU'RE THE HOSTESS

When you want to be the hostess with the mostess, assign someone (a sanguine or "I" personality type is best for this) the job of being the official greeter. Inform the greeter of the names of guests so that he or she can greet them personally. Having name tags is a debatable subject, but it's usually an effective way to help everyone when it's a blended crowd of people who do not formally know each other and also when the group is larger than ten.

Having beverages easily accessible is a must; offer a variety of options for your guests' comfort. If serving alcohol, always offer an option for those who do not prefer it. The hostess's main job is to mingle with guests and provide a pleasant experience for them. When you are confident with your appearance, you are more apt to give honest attention to others and make them feel special. It's a great idea to have someone else serving food and drinks (if it's that kind of party) so that the hostess can host.

Exchanging business cards with flair is something I learned from my dad when I was in high school. Although embarrassing at the time, I now know it to be a valuable lesson: always hand out two or three cards at a time, one for the immediate recipient and one or two for him or her to pass on. Asking for a card first usually prompts someone to ask for yours and makes the exchange natural. The best way to connect quickly through conversation in a business setting is to ask questions, find a commonality, and then engage. Use the other person's name often during conversation, as it will help you remember him or her later. I often write a few key words or our common interests right on the back of the card as soon as possible because it helps me remember the person when I get back to my office.

As with everything in life, there are exceptions to these business etiquette rules. Adapt to the nature of the business and the setting. The easiest example I can give is one that we handle on a regular basis. My husband is a home builder in a small town. It's not unusual for a business function to be a barbecue social in a country barn, with picnic tables and bales of straw nearby. This is a lot different from attending a business function in downtown Orlando at a high-end venue. You get the idea. The nature of your business influences the formalities you should follow. Some folks call it "situational awareness." It's basically being aware of your surroundings, relating well to others, and, for the purposes of this book, being appropriately dressed. And to that latter point, if you're unsure, dress one step up rather than one step down. The barbecue attire doesn't mean, however, that you can't wear rhinestone belts, bling earrings, and jewel-studded jeans. Have some fun if only to impress yourself.

This is obviously not a chapter on complete social graces, but knowing some basics will help you improve your confidence so that nothing will detract from all your efforts to dress for success!

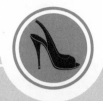

STEP UP TO ACTION:

Shop 'til Ya Drop?

Do you frequently shop at small, local boutiques, larger retail chains and online? If not, commit to trying a shop that you've never been in before.

To keep yourself from falling victim to the allure of a sale price over value and need, ask whether the item can be worn at least three different ways, with three different items you already have and for more than one season.

The word that best describes my fashion preference is:.

_____

N2K recommendation: When there's a discrepancy on what to wear to an event, always go with the dressier option. "Casual" on an invitation usually means that a man need not come in a coat and tie.

Chapter 8

ACCESSORIZE TO MAXIMIZE

"The only thing that separates us from the animals is the ability to accessorize."

—*Robert Harling,* **Steel Magnolias**

If you feel like a birdbrain when it comes to knowing how to accessorize, you'll be ready to put on the dogs after you read this chapter. With a little courage to step out boldly and try new things, you'll begin to develop a signature style all your own. Accessories have indeed been THE item that can take your look from good to great in a moment and have you strutting like a peacock on your way out the door!

The ability to accessorize can also separate us from the pack so that our message gets through all the noise; why settle for a meek "meow" when your image could "roar" before you even say a word? To do that, most of us can benefit from a few tips about how to use accessories to complete our head-to-toe look. Much the way that adding the right frame to any work of art helps the viewer appreciate it more, so can adding the right finishing touches to something as simple as the LBD—little black dress—turn it from a basic, looks-good-on-everybody black sheath into an embellished, mouth-dropping, stunning, wearable piece of art. (This is such a classic piece. . . . You do have at least one hanging in your closet, right?) Even if your goal isn't to turn heads, you can still create a statement and pull together a finished form that says "chic" rather than "yawn."

Of course, accessories aren't just for the LDB; they are the finishing touches on every outfit. In the last chapter, we learned about which style options would best complement your personality. Here, we'll focus on completing the look you're going for, from Boho or traditional Talbots to vintage or Victorian or even to a retro street fashion that reaches globally. The same principle applies—part of your daily wardrobe essentials should include at least one of the following to emphasize your personal style: necklace, earrings, bracelet, hair clip, ring, scarf, hat, glasses, purse, belt, stockings, or shoes. They easily and affordably update your look, much the way changing out pillows updates the look in your home. And please note that "complementing" doesn't always mean matching, which was popular for the past two decades (although you're not considered completely out of style if your purse and shoes *do* match).

Knowing which accessories look best on you and with each outfit can take a little practice. Just because a trend is in doesn't mean it's in for you, and just because something is considered "classic" doesn't mean you can't jazz it up to match your look. For example, Barbara Bush will always be remembered for her classic use of pearls. They just "fit" her. If you like pearls but love the Boho look, find ways to incorporate pearls in other ways, such as a funky pin or bodacious buttons. As you select from a smorgasbord of accessories, make sure you stay true to what "fits" you. Employ the same basic principles already laid out for color recommendations to bring out your best. Use accessories to the max; just be careful not to miss the mark.

Know, first, who you are; and then adorn yourself accordingly.

—Epictetus

SENDING THE RIGHT VIBE

Marilyn Monroe used to look in the mirror when she would leave the house and remove whatever piece of jewelry she noticed first. Why? Because she wanted others to notice HER, not her clothing or jewelry. She adhered to this principle from head to toe, and I believe it's a principle worthy of our attention. You see, while the right accessories can totally make the outfit, the wrong ones can be a total distraction. Imagine . . .

you're trying to have a conversation with a potential client, but she can't concentrate on what you're saying because all your bangle bracelets are clanging, or she's calculating the price of so much bling, or maybe she's wondering how you don't have a neck ache with all the chains you're wearing. While we're on the subject, I might as well mention that too many holes for rings in various parts of your body is most certainly a distraction for the majority of the population and never appropriate for a job interview. Moderation is key, as is the occasion you are dressing for. You would do well to wear more conservative jewelry to a job interview than a night on the town. You get the idea. When in doubt, a good rule of thumb is to use one great piece to create a focal point.

A focal point could be a bold, colorful purse for a big pop of color; a flowing scarf that seems to pull your top and bottom together; or a wide leather belt with rhinestones for a sassy, biker-chic look. Whatever piece you use, realize this is your biggest wardrobe investment and where you'll get the best bang for your buck. Mix metals; the combination of silver and gold is often much more sophisticated than one metal alone (if it still makes you nervous, invest in one necklace or bracelet that incorporates both metals; this piece will "marry" your solid gold and silver pieces and help them to play nice).

PERSONAL EXPRESSION: TRENDY OR CLASSIC?

Determining whether your personal style preference is more trendy/ eclectic or classic/modern will help you stay in line with that same theme for accessorizing. Whether you're a jewelry lover or not, you must make sure you have these essentials. **A trendy look** includes bling rings, bunches of bangles, hoop earrings, and lots of chunky, tribal chains, short or long. **A classic look** includes a simple pendent necklace such as classic pearls or diamonds, stud earrings, one or two rings (in addition to your wedding ring, if you wear one), and either one bracelet and watch or a functional and fun belt. And if you're not a jewelry lover, you might find your signature mark to be more easily made through wearing stylish belts, shoes, eyeglasses, or hair accessories or even by the use of business items such as funky pens, leopard (or any theme) datebooks, file folders, notebooks, key chains, and so on. I haven't mentioned all the possible choices and ways you can accessorize, but I've given enough examples for you to move in a direction that helps you define your personal style. It's just one more way to stand out in the crowd.

In the same way that we will soon learn to do with body shapes and clothing selection, we can use accessories to maximize our best feature and minimize our trouble spots. Is your best asset your face, your waist, your longer legs, or your hands? For example, if you are blessed to have an hourglass figure, you can easily wear belts cinched at the waist. If your body shape is a petite apple, you're better off wearing long necklaces and drop earrings, thus creating vertical lines. Short, nubby fingers with unkempt nails do not need to be wearing big bling rings. A woman with a longer neck can create the illusion of "filling in the space" between her face and body with a choker or a bold necklace that falls just at the neckline and a bigger round style of earring that adds width and depth. Petite body shapes call for petite jewelry; be careful not to overpower. Larger body shapes with a less than flat middle can wear all sorts of big, bold jewelry, especially on the upper part of the body. And if there's one piece of jewelry everyone can wear and should have, it's a cocktail ring!

Wearing a cocktail ring gives you that "diva" feeling and look. Maybe that's why they're so popular among celebrities. Cocktail rings are often candy colored, cute, or glittering and glamorous and use all kinds of gems and semiprecious stones such as corals, turquoise, garnets, and pearls. The chunky rings can make a simple, elegant statement or a very bold and high-impact one. They aren't as pricey as they often look, making it easy for fashionistas to jazz up their jewelry dreams without breaking the bank. Cocktail rings with faux stones range in price from as little as $15 to a few hundred dollars and can be found everywhere accessories are, from Tiffany's and Zales to QVC including handmade and custom pieces; there are endless alternatives to every kind of jewelry you will ever want.

Costume jewelry is really all the rave right now, and celebs are helping to create thriving businesses for direct-sales companies. Color is a key component, and it's always interesting what inspires designers—everything from architecture to vintage. Art Deco–inspired collar necklaces and large but surprisingly light angular-shaped earrings that instantly dress up basics and show up like real sparklers in paparazzi and red-carpet pictures are everywhere. Costume jewelry is a fantastic way to update your style with a little bit (or plenty) of ooomph and spice! Bring on the bangles, please . . . One is simply not enough.

Fashion hats range from classy, trendy fedoras to wide-brim sun hats. Whichever style you choose, a hat can considerably modify your look because it changes the size and appearance of your head. Each person has to decide whether that's an improvement or not! Some are worn for fashion alone, and others are for shielding from the elements, whether sun or chill. A hat can emphasize a round face, shorten a long face, balance out a bottom-heavy body shape, or make you look like an ice cream cone. **A hat can make or break your look**. Your choice of hat and how you wear it will automatically brand you as stylish or style-less. It basically sends an instant message of who you are, and those around you will definitely notice! Since your face is the first thing people do notice about you, a hat will intensify your first impression. If being a little "out there" is something you want to portray, this is one accessory to help you do just that. We have the wide-brim hats that scream glam and style, fedoras that give you a cool and sexy look, and berets that add a cute feel to your outfit. Each and every hat type already sends a strong message of who you are; wearing them with class is a fun way to express that.

Scarves, like hats, are a quick way to alter an outfit and add a pop of style without overdoing it. And they're quite versatile and practical when it's cold, either outside or in an overly air-conditioned space. Scarves can help separate the color between your neck and your face so that your best colors are used to introduce your face. They can also create a more fluid look with monochromatic tones if that is a better adjustment. You can quickly grab a scarf as you are dashing out the door to school or work and not worry much whether it matches. A scarf can help cover some cleavage, too, which can be especially useful for women in business situations, where there should be no confusing a boardroom with a bedroom.

From a fashion sense, they come in every style to complete the perfect outfit: pashmina wool, cotton, lace, silk, chiffon, blended, leopard, or vintage. My favorite use of the silk style is under a suit jacket that I wear often but find in warm climates to be uncomfortably hot. A slinky tank for coolness and a fashionable scarf are the perfect answer to my dilemma. This achieves my goal of making a fashion statement with the scarf and also gives me comfort options for wearing the suit year-round. The best part about scarves is that a single one can be worn a dozen different ways. I recommend getting at least one in a neutral tone that will serve you from casual to business for a long time to come.

Having even one scarf-tying trick in your bag gives you a little alternative to the same old guise, so here it is: the pleated drape. Take an oblong scarf and tie a very loose knot on one side of the scarf just a few inches from the end. Drape it around your neck so that the two ends are hanging evenly in front. Take the unknotted side and accordion pleat it from the end up about seven inches. Let go of the pleats in one hand and hold them in the other as you slide the pleats halfway through the knot. This will complete the circle around your neck as you pull the knot tight and fan out the pleats. I usually wear the "pleated bow" off-centered and sometimes pin it from underneath to hold in place. For a video tutorial on this and other scarf-tying tricks, visit www.NakedtoKnockout.com. Other versions include a simple bow, using a rubber band to create a faux bow, the classic knot, the slipknot, and the ascot wrap. You can use scarves as head coverings, around your neck tightly as a necklace, as a belt, and certainly as shawls and coat wraps. Versatility to the max!

Handbags are the absolute wardrobe necessity for every woman of any age. Come on, what else is going to stylishly carry your essentials? The style range includes small evening clutches, hobo bags, tote bags, designer bags, briefcases, and every kind of purse you could crave. Adding a red patent leather bag to a monochromatic navy blue outfit makes a stellar statement! Denim capris with a citrus block-colored top may call for a structured boxy-style bag or even a smaller floral patterned clutch on a chain. An organic neutral skirt and sweater with a fun, frilly, vintage Boho-style bag draped across your front serves as a perfectly functional accessory, too.

On handbags, I'm often asked how I organize them all. Besides having custom closets recently built, I recommend you go to sites such as Get Organized, www.orgbydesignonline.com, or www.Organize.com or refer to Lorie Marrero, professional organizer, at www.clutterdiet.com. When you have a collection of purses for every outfit and every occasion, the problem of storage is most likely a major concern in your closet, too. I love the canvas hanging purse organizer that holds ten purses and provides a quick and easy way to store and organize your handbags and free up space in your cluttered closet.

Another cool little tool is a purse organizer, sold by a variety of companies. It provides a place to keep all your essentials, and you can easily pull out just that one insert to put in the next bag when you make a change. If you're like me, asking my husband to grab my purse is like sending him to the grocery store for some fruit. He never knows which one I'm referring to. Maybe the confusion also comes from the fact that there's usually one on my car's front seat, one in my office, one on the bedroom chair, and one hanging near the back door. Oh, my, I think I need to call Lorie!

ON YOUR MARK, GET SET, GO!

Look in a full-length mirror from head to toe and see whether there is harmony. Does your look seem choppy or fluid? Do the accessories complement or compete? Be objective enough to ask yourself what message you get when you see others dressed like you. Based on appearance, would you be attracted to you? Start small if you need to; even one image update will get you headed on the road to success. Hiring an image consultant will take the guesswork out and save you time and money in the long run. Plus, we know where all the really good deals are, so it makes for even more time- and money-saving benefits on your end! With a consultant, we begin a thorough assessment of what you have I your closet, what you don't need, what you do need, and what your goals are. I will give you an action plan and steps for improving your image that can be implemented immediately. If you are concerned about what to wear to a big event such as a class reunion, wedding, cruise, speaking engagement, print or media opportunity, or black-tie dinner event, I can help you with a consultation for that as well. You will benefit from the free download e-version of my style guide that recaps these tips and more . . . It's perfect to have on your phone. Simply sign in on my **website: www.NakedtoKnockout.com** and get yours today!

Clothes help us celebrate who we are, and the final touches we add help define and advertise our personal message. Last, I would be remiss not to mention the value of the least expensive, most accessible asset of all. Flash those pearly whites and turn that frown upside down. Cliché, I know. But it's true; a smile is the best, most visible, most important accessory. No animal necklace, friendship bracelet, or hand-knit scarf conjures up the beauty and connection that a smile does. If you leave the house in an outfit that's chic, interesting, and accessorized, people will look at you. When they do, smile at them! It thrills the friendly and disarms the smug. If they're already admiring what you're wearing and then you look like a nice person on top of it, they might even muster the nerve to compliment you—and that makes everyone feel good.

Wearing accessories appropriately is like adorning gift wrap. They can be utilized to create desire for what's inside. Inviting others to unwrap the gift of YOU and truly engage begins with an initial great first impression. You can do it with class and style!

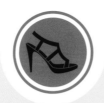

Look in the Mirror and Like what you see!

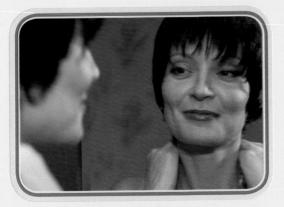

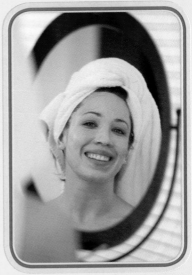

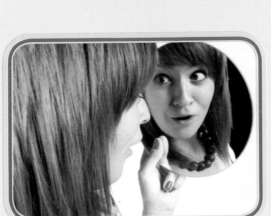

It all begins with the way YOU view yourself! Being sexy in your own skin is sometimes a process of learning how to take yourself off the discount rack and display your extraordinary self! Remember to tell yourself daily that YOU HAVE VALUE AND YOU MATTER when you look in the mirror.

Mirror, Mirror on the wall, Who's the fairest of them all? Golly, gee it must be me ... 'cuz I'm the only one I see!

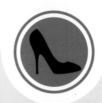

Color Confidence!

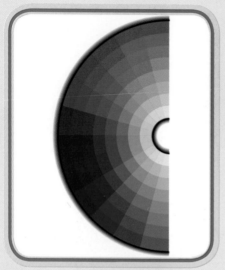

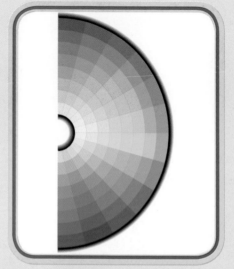

COOL color collection: also common for Summer and Winter tones. Colors with blue undertones

WARM color collection: also common for Spring and Fall tones. Colors with yellow undertones

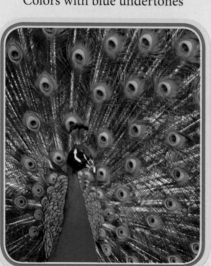

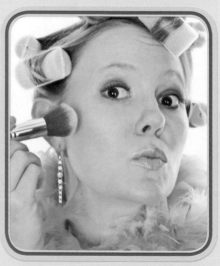

When you're wearing your knockout colors, you'll be prancing like a peacock.

Becoming color confident takes a little practice but is not hard! Throw on a boa and have fun.

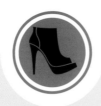

Glamour Glitz!

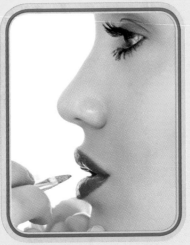

Any finished product gives attention to the canvas. Start fresh with a good skin care regime and add all the glitz you want to suit your mood and desired result. From an every day "Dash out the Door" look to a natural, classic and business look, to a dramatic evening allure one ... this is the place to express your personality to the fullest.

N2K principle for optimum results:

Use the right colors
Use the right tools
Use the right technique

Congrats!
You're on your way
to knockout status!

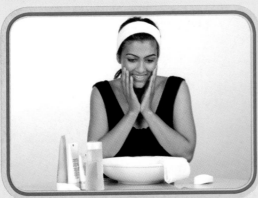

"You can take no credit for beauty at sixteen but if you are beautiful at sixty, it will be your soul's own doing."

—Marie Stopes

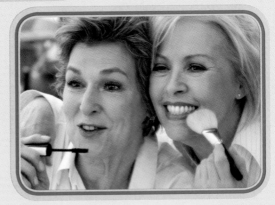

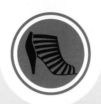

Dress for Success

KNOWING YOUR SEASON HELPS YOU SHOP "ON PURPOSE" – refer to page 45

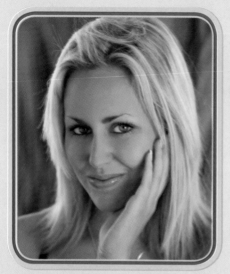

Here's a classy, sassy
SUMMER.

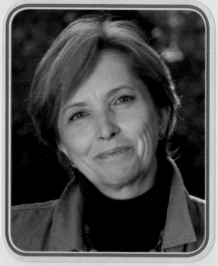

Here's an amazing
AUTUMN

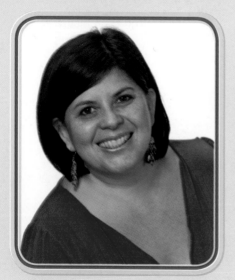

Here's a wonderful
WINTER

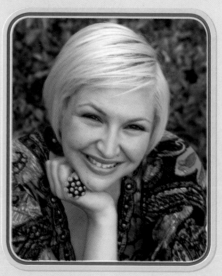

Here's a spectacular
SPRING

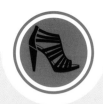

Accessories: The perfect finishing touch

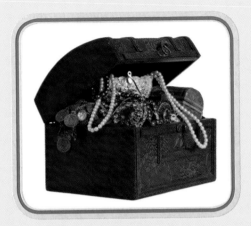

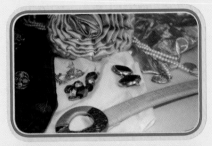

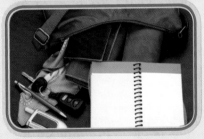

Accessories ... think of them as your treasure chest for creating new looks from existing pieces. They include business accessories, shoes, scarves, jewelry, belts, hats, purses, pins—this is where your personal style can shine! Adding a pop of color or one statement piece can take a drab outfit and make it FAB.

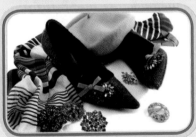

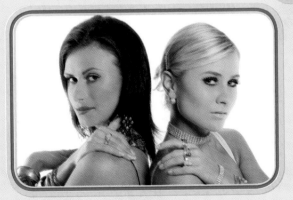

Mixing metals is always an option. These women are examples of a WINTER and SUMMER model in both gold and silver jewelry ... Black or white ... it's always a classic look.

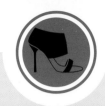

Got chaos in your closet?

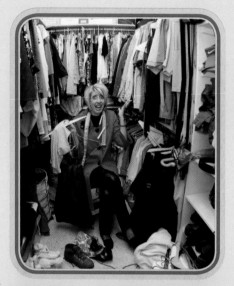

Please, no wire hangers. The wooden ones are far better. We shot these before and after pictures during our closet makeover before it aired as a show: "Coming out of your closet in style." My main rule: Have a place for everything and everything in its place. Bins and tubs to sort items for giveaway, throw away, or simple organizing will help de-clutter in a practical and visual way. Use clear ones so that you can always see what's inside each container. Stack shoes together ... always. Enjoy your morning routine!

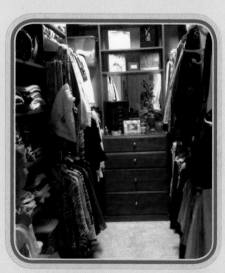

"However beautiful the strategy, you should occasionally look at the results".

—Winston Churchill

Photos courtesy of
Healthy Living Magazine

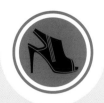

Creating a style all your own . . .

Individual creativity starts with the realization that you are created as a Unique U! Become style solution oriented. Wear a smile. Have on one great piece of jewelry. Get a slammin' hair do. Treat yourself to a mani and pedi. Change your lipstick color. Dress to flatter your figure. Lean on your strengths. Honor yourself. Take a tiny step out of your comfort zone. Whatever your style, embrace the inner and outer beauty of you!

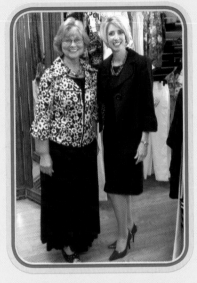

At the boutique doing some personalized shopping with a client.

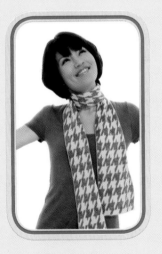

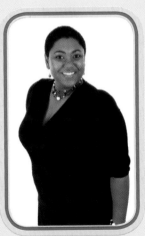

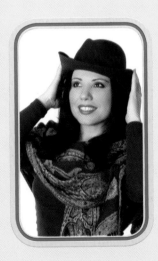

"If honor be your clothing, the suit will last a lifetime; but if clothing be your honor, it will soon be worn threadbare"

—William Arnot

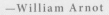

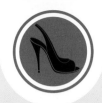

Wendy Lyn Phillips

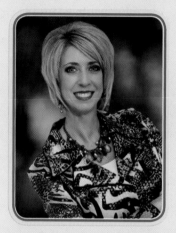

. . . is a professional image and beauty expert. She combines 25 years of experience in the beauty industry consulting thousands of women to help them create a more compelling and confident presence As an entrepreneur for all of her adult life, Wendy Lyn has inspired many to step up their personal and professional style. She has reached the top 5% in sales and leadership nationwide with her company for the last 15 years. She is a dynamic speaker that teaches N2Kworkshops and believes every woman deserves to look in the mirror and like what she sees. As an expert in relating to working moms, Wendy Lyn knows the value of being able to "Dash out the Door" and do it, in style. She is also becoming known as the "speakers" consultant—assisting professional speakers and business owners to ensure their image reflects their message. Wendy is also a monthly contributor to many magazines and has been a guest on numerous national radio and local TV stations. This "Chic mom" of 2 young girls resides in central Florida where she and her husband are enjoying their excitement-packed, surprises-occurring-daily, fun-filled and blessed life. You'll find her enjoying time with them, her church and her community when she's not traveling.

Find us on Facebook, Twitter, LinkedIn, and enjoy her weekly Knockout blog. Visit our website to book her for an INNERgizing keynote speaking engagement, a workshop with your organization, personal image coaching or emceeing your next event.

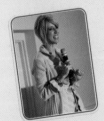
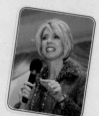
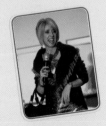
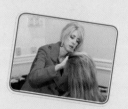

Pictures compliments of Malcolm Yawn—**www.malcolmyawn.com**.

Find out more at: www.NakedtoKnockout.com

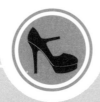

STEP UP TO ACTION:
Your Wardrobe Storyboard

Take pictures of your outfit "sets" with shoes and all accessories and make a storyboard. When you have that special event you're convinced you have nothing to wear to, the storyboard will help you remember the great combinations that you do have.

• It will also keep you from forgetting the impressive collection of accessories that you've accumulated. (If you're like me, "out of sight, out of mind"!)

• It enables you to pack quickly for your next trip.

• It takes the guesswork out of always having to re-create an outfit. Go with what you know looks great, feels great and fits. (Refer to Mitzi Purdue's recommendation in chapter 2.)

What one accessory is your best statement piece?

What one accessory would you most like to start incorporating into your style?

Chapter 9

DOES WHAT'S IN YOUR CLOSET LIKE YOU?

Why is it that most American women have closets full of clothes but the first thing we say when we open the door is "I have nothing to wear!"? It is sad. And once you rummage through all the "nothings" in the closet, how many times do you hear yourself say, "Does this outfit make me look fat?"

What if you could put on clothes every day and love what you saw in the mirror? Pure bliss, right? Are you tired of going through three outfit changes before you feel good enough to walk out the door? I can relate. My four-year-old is now up to an average of 7.5 changes a day! I swear I had nothing to do with it. I'm not sure whether it's because she's unsettled about her fashion decisions, because she loves clothes so much (and has too many), or because there is some serious attention deficit disorder forming in her.

Seriously, though, Americans are bombarded with shopping frenzy experiences on a daily basis: sales, deals, thrift shop options, online instant purchasing, next-day delivery (with free returns), marketing jingles, and high-end gotta-haves! Women usually love what they buy yet hate two-thirds of what's in their closets. When exactly does the disconnect happen? When did "I love this new outfit I just purchased" suddenly change to "I hate what's in my closet"?

Maybe it's time to ask, "Does what's in my closet like me?" Are they the right shades of green for my autumn needs . . . Are there buttons that need replacing . . . hems too long or short . . . Do they hang right without bunching in places . . . Do my clothes like me because they actually fit me and make me feel like a knockout when I wear them? Learning to come out of your closet in style starts with what's IN your closet, and loving what's IN there is possible.

Feeling WOW after getting dressed on a daily basis takes mental discipline, some "know how to flatter your figure" basics, and a few fashion faux pas to avoid. Being sexy in your own skin is an attitude but looking sophisticated can certainly take some knack. It starts with making good shopping choices so that you like what's in your closet AND what's in your closet also likes you (your body shape).

Confident of what colors look the most complementary ON you and the styles that are most appropriate FOR you takes a lot of the guesswork out of the shopping experience. If the piece is a style you love but not in your right color, do not purchase it! Likewise, if it's something in a color you love but is too tight or too loose, the same principle goes: do not purchase. And we all know that the hardest thing to avoid is the sale dilemma: but it's ON SALE! It's a steal! Well, don't make a big deal about a good deal if it makes you look like, well, you know. Those bargain-buying boo-boos pile up, and trust me, there's no pony hiding underneath them! That sale item is a lot more costly than you think if the item rarely gets worn. It also costs you time spent taking it on and off trying to make it work when it shouldn't even be in your closet in the first place. Worse yet is that no matter what it costs, if it just stays in your closet and you never get any wear out of it, how much of a savings was that, really? Time to donate.

Knockout Know-How

There are two main reasons women don't dress for success: we think it's expensive and we simply don't know how. The right wardrobe is not difficult to accumulate, and it doesn't have to be expensive. The most important thing to understand so you can avoid buying boo-boos is to know what is right for you and what is not. There are many factors that play into this decision. We have become such a quick-fix society that we don't often think about purchases properly. Before buying, train yourself to answer the following questions; if you can't answer YES to at least two of them, the purchase is off:

- Do I need it? Or, if it's a "want," is it in my price point budget?
- Can I wear it at least three different ways: (1) casually, (2) for work, and (3) combined with something else for a formal affair?
- Is it the right color for me?
- Is it the right style for my body shape?

Two out of four yeses make it a strong purchase possibility in my book. This little quiz has kept me from falling victim to buying on impulse and then getting home to feel guilty and asking myself, "Why did I get this again?" or "What I am going to wear that with?" Making a purchase that was a great deal, a great fit, and a great color is a GREAT THING! And, after reading and referring to my handy style guide for business dress, you will both **FEEL like a knockout AND LOOK like one, too**! Make sure you get one to drop in your purse and refer to while shopping.

GO FIGURE

Liking what you see in the mirror gets a whole lot easier once you understand how to make the best choices for YOUR figure rather than letting a random sale price or anonymous clerk tempt you into buying what's not in your best fashion interest. Knowing your figure type will make it easy to figure out what to buy. The trick is sticking to it even when you are tempted. Remember the basics: if you're shorter and fuller, creating vertical lines is your goal. If you're leaner or taller (even full figure with height), horizontal lines and bolder prints are for you. Most all women benefit from drawing attention away from their "less than flat" middle. Create balance and focal points near your face with a slamming hairdo, impeccable makeup, jewelry adequately placed, and great shoes always. *Don't pay any attention to the number for sizing on tags; its only purpose is to help you know which ones to take into the dressing room and try on.*

EVERY body shape is special because it houses a very unique, one-of-a-kind person—YOU!

Let's start by reinforcing the types of clothing that best flatter your figure by defining the five main body types. I like to refer to them in shapes: the triangle, the circle, the rectangle, the hourglass (double triangle), and the petite. Now, it can get a little fruity when you start recognizing the pears, apples, and bananas in the mirror. So as not to become a basket case, remember that every fruit has a certain benefit, color, and value!

IT'S REALLY EASY TO FIGURE OUT

*TRIANGLES (or pears) are wider on the bottom than the top. It's all about drawing the eye up and creating BALANCE. To look your best:

- Consider color's power: bring the eye up by keeping patterns or bright colors on top; minimize attention on the hips by using single darker colors from your waist down.

- Broaden your shoulders with tops that have wider necklines such as scoop necks or open collars. Shoulder pads can help, but keep them to a minimum.

- Jackets should stop just above the widest part of the hip; look for shawl or wider collars.

- Choose skirts with an A-line or straight styling, such as pencil skirts; avoid pleats or gathers at the waist.

- Choose dresses such as empire cuts or A-line styles. An embellished neckline or straps keep the attention above the hips.

- Avoid pants with tapered legs (the "ice cream cone" effect).

- Avoid patterned trousers or jeans with lots of fading on the rear and thighs. The boot-cut-style jean usually works well.

*CIRCLES (or apples/plus sizes) are curvaceous. It's all about sculpting those curves and defining the waist. To look your best:

- Consider color's power: dark solid colors will make the figure look smaller, as will dressing in the same color. Skip the trendy all-over, oversized-patterned fabrics, but do feel free to add a splash of color near the face to draw the eye up.

- Single-breasted jackets are most flattering, with a tailored, structured style and V neckline. If you are short, look for jackets that stop at the hip so you don't look even shorter. Avoid pockets at the hips; look for asymmetrical closings for a more slimming effect.

- Skirts should hover around the knee, just above or below, and should have a narrow profile (no gathering, ruffles, or unstitched pleats) in a soft, flowing fabric.

- Note that shapeless clothing adds weight but structured styles add shape and are visually slimming.

- Avoid heavy fabrics and the ones that cling to all the wrong places.

- Avoid tight fits. Sit, bend, and move around as you would on a normal day and see how the garment fits. The bust, armholes, and torso on tops/ jackets and the hips/backside on skirts and pants should not pinch, restrict movement, or gape open.

- SPANX are a must!

*RECTANGLES (or bananas/straight/boyish) do not have an obvious waistline or hips. It's all about adding definition and creating or maximizing what curves are there. To look your best:

- Consider color's power: strong colors and patterns add fullness to your hips.

- Jackets that nip in at the waist and add a flare at the hipline work well. Think peplums, wrap styles that tie or belt at the waist and flare out, and double-breasted styles that are well structured to create curves. Avoid short, boxy jackets that stop at the waist.

- Choose skirts that add fullness, such as sarongs and trumpet skirts.
- Choose tops or dresses with some ruching for a curvy effect. Square necklines with a fitted waist add more structure and shape.
- Avoid clingy, flimsy fabrics and high-waisted pants or skirts.
- Avoid vertical stripes and patterns, which diminish curves and make you look lanky.

*HOURGLASSES (larger at top and hips with small waist) need to work at proportion control by accentuating their best feature, their smaller middle. To look your best:

- Consider color's power: use monochromatic tones or the same hue sweater or jacket at the top as the bottom and a black shell/tank (which is really the "go-to" look for most all of the body shapes).
- Business suit jackets should be classic cuts with one or two buttons; for casual jackets, go with short denim. Drop-waisted coats are a no-no.
- Try dresses with cinched middles or wraps. The sheath style is especially great for work.
- Wear wide belts to accentuate the smaller waist.
- Wear structured clothing such as tops with lines, a square neck, and fitted button-under-the-bust blazers or cardigans. Unless you're petite, bold accessories are very good.
- Ruffles can help create a V line at the neck and are fine on a skirt bottom for a feminine flair.
- Pants that are flared or cuffed are best.
- Jeans look FAB in a boot cut.

*PETITES (5'4" or under) In general, your goal is to shop for vertical lines, monochromatic colors, choose v-necklines, smaller prints and soft, fluid, lightweight fabrics. Divide the petite figure at uneven points with short-over-long or long-over-short silhouettes. Refrain from making the figure look shorter by cutting it in half. Keep the attention toward the upper body for added height.

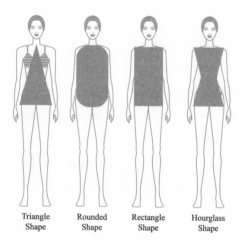

| Triangle Shape | Rounded Shape | Rectangle Shape | Hourglass Shape |

For all figure types, it helps to find a good tailor who can tweak a garment to fit you perfectly! Utilize a personal shopper when available, as most all big department stores have them. (At the back of the book I have included other resources whose Web sites you can peruse.) Another consideration is to stick with accentuating the shape you are today, not the shape you wish you were, used to be, or someday hope to be. Don't hide your shape behind a muumuu unless you are in your thirty-ninth week of pregnancy! Accept and present your shape in a way that is both comfortable and attractive! It IS possible for clothing to be both.

WARDROBE MULTIPLICATION

I am a strong proponent of creating mix-and-match options with your clothing, and this starts by having an organized closet that makes it easier to find the items you want. One way to do this is to buy separate suit components, whether pantsuits, skirted ones, or other "like" outfits that you commonly bought together. When you get home, separate them and hang each piece in different parts of your closet. Hang all your tops together, business attire in one section, and casual in another, and group your pants, skirts, jackets, and formals. Another great organizing and wardrobe-multiplying tip I learned from a friend is to put the newest, fresh-out-of-the-dryer clothing at the back of your rack and take the item you are going to wear today from the front end (i.e., left to right). This helps in two ways: first, you don't waste time trying to remember whether you already wore that top to work this week and, second, you quickly see whether there are items that have been at the front of the rack all year. If so, it's time to give them away to a friend, sell them on eBay or at an upscale consignment store, or else donate them to a charity! If it's something you really love and it's a style that you simply don't wear that often, it is OK to keep it, but that should be the exception to the rule, which is: *if it hasn't been worn at least once in the past year, it's time to consider recycling.*

Again, the best way to get a handle on this is to get your closet organized. You'd be amazed at how much easier it is to get dressed for the day once you do it. I recently had the privilege of working with ORG by Design to produce a Web TV show that resulted in my getting a totally new custom closet makeover. It has completely transformed my morning routine. I just love what a new closet makeover by ORG by Design has done to reduce my getting-dressed dilemmas; you'll love what they can do for you, too!

Perhaps it's time to revisit the system you have in place for keeping an updated, organized closet. *You do have a system, don't you?* For example, "one in, one out," which means that for each new item you buy, you let one go. Or maybe you have one or more "someday" piles, as in "Someday I'll wear this after I lose ten pounds" or "Someday this will come back in style." Piling up the piles leads to closet chaos, and that makes it hard to find the pony hiding underneath it all. Here are five things that you can do today to tame the chaos in your closet:

1. Use the same type of hangers for everything. Whether it's wood, plastic, or metal, find a kind that you prefer and stick to it. The visual effect of your clothes hanging the same length, the same way, gives an instant appearance of organization. And please get rid of any wire hangers that no longer hold their shape!

2. Go vertical by using all the wall space. There is normally wasted space above the top shelf. If you have room, install additional shelving where extra space is not being used. Home improvement stores have shelving often under $20 that can double your storage space for items that aren't worn as frequently.

3. Use bins and baskets to store items such as out-of-season clothing, baseball caps, purses, belts, and scarves.

4. Keep baskets or bins in your closet for items that you'd like to DONATE or SELL. I already mentioned the "one in, one out" system, which is a good place to start, but let's take it a step further. Ask yourself, *Can I give it away? Do I need to sell it? Do I need to throw it away?* Make your three piles and get going! Having containers that are labeled for these items will keep everything in its place. Once the bin is labeled, I don't have to "think" about the items anymore and have it be an emotional decision. Just do it!

5. As for the "someday . . . " system, chances are that by the time you are ready to wear it again, the style or colors will have changed and you will want something new. It's best to free up the closet space now so you will have room for the clothes you love and want to wear today. Be a blessing to others and just get rid of your "someday" pile. Carpe diem!

(*Some data printed from Laura Leist with permission, 2011; www. eliminatechaos.com*)

CARRY ON

Packing light for travel is not my specialty, and in my business, I've traveled a lot, and that's put a great deal of stress on my shoulders—literally. I have learned from some really talented people how to do this more effectively and efficiently.

Packing smart to reduce stress is appealing, and anyone can learn how. I am proud to say that on my recent four-day business trip to New

York City, I achieved what I once believed was impossible: one carry-on and one extra oversized bag that served as my purse. Hoorah for me! And, yup, that means all my makeup and personal items were in legal travel size, my five pairs of shoes had jewelry and undergarments stuffed in them, and my outfits were strategically decided beforehand with packing light in mind. My husband will tell you I have come a loooong way since our honeymoon, when I lugged along three extra-large suitcases and two carry-ons. Excuse me; *he* was the pack mule lugging all the baggage. True love for sure. So, yes, there's hope. My hardest packing decisions come from uncertainty about the weather. It's often warm outside but freezing inside convention meeting places. Plus, the weather changes, as does my mood. Solution: be logical and pack a black sweater, jacket, or sassy raincoat. Then there are the spontaneous events that occur where I have wished I had other articles with me.

All of these are good things to consider when attempting to pack light *and* thorough. Savvy travelers create a packing list for each trip. This will help you be on purpose when packing as well as provide for a checklist that you can use over and over; when you return, make notes on that list, such as "great travel pants" or "wrinkled terribly" or "never wore" so you remember what worked and what did not. For me, it's usually a decision of what shoes can I wear that are both comfy and cute. This answers many of my what-to-wear-dilemmas . . . especially during travel. If you are traveling for a speaking engagement, attending special events, or making presentations to groups, you may want to note on your calendar what you wore on each trip so as to not repeat it. While the LBD is a great investment, you don't want to see yourself wearing it in every picture at every charity event. When packing for a new trip, review the lists, make the adjustments based on your notes, and see whether your packing-induced stress doesn't just disappear. Don't depend on recall, the faintest ink is better than the most retentive memory!

DRESS WITH YOUR DESTINATION IN MIND

An added dimension to feeling WOW as you leave your closet is to acknowledge your purpose and destination; be sure to consider what message your look is conveying and its appropriateness for where you're going.

For instance, overdressing can be just as detrimental as underdressing. You especially want to consider the difference your jewelry can make to dress an outfit up or down. What you might wear with a classic black Traveler collection from Chico's in the day can easily turn into an evening look with a quick change and added glitz. Just be careful not to overdo it during the daytime . . . It could keep others at a distance and thinking you're unapproachable. This same idea goes for almost any business suit that is meant for the office during daytime but can easily be "reaccessorized" for evening.

Dressing too casual or worse can be just as detrimental for keeping others at a distance. Just recently, a client asked for some fashion help because her friend finally told her that her style looked too "ghetto." Hence, the call came to me. It is always fascinating to me how women can be involved in community, business, and social circles without giving at least some serious attention to the message their appearance conveys. We simply get so busy in the daily flow of life or stay so focused on what we are doing that we inadvertently settle for looking "just good enough" to get by. We've all dashed out of the house looking disheveled, with every intention of just running a couple of errands, thinking that we'd "really get dressed" once we got home. And isn't it that very day you see just the person you are embarrassed to have seen you? We've all had that happen.

I can't help but reinforce the simple solution we all can implement to prevent that from happening: take a few seconds to look in the mirror before leaving the house. After spending time and energy on learning how to LIKE what you see (your inner beauty), take the time and energy to LOOK IN THE MIRROR! I think of Marilyn Monroe again; she would take one last look in the mirror before she dashed out the door. So, ladies, hang a mirror near the door you frequent the most!

This reminds me of a time in my life when my "closet" was literally in my trunk. Yep, three large garbage bags for my most frequently worn clothes. Now mind you, I was in college, it was summer and I lived near the beach, and it was a transitional time when I was living with a friend. My three bags helped me stay organized: one included my swim suits, cute cover ups, shirts and shorts, the other was my work clothes and the other was for lingerie. My sundresses and anything else that needed to be hung, was . . . in the back seat of my car. I will never forget the simplicity of having a few basics that I felt very confident in wearing on a rare date or out with friends. It really is better to have fewer, high quality items that work for you. The funny part is I recently found some of those classic items and sold them to a consignment . . . yes, twenty years later! When you buy classic styles that hold up and aren't too trendy, you can do that.

Our closets can be tiny spaces that hold only the essentials for daily covering the trunk of your car, or walk-in rooms full of every organizing bin and basket imaginable, complete with cherry wood trim and crown molding. Regardless of your physical space, view it as a design arena that prepares you to face the world each day. Since getting dressed is a daily chore, make it one you enjoy by loving what's in your closet AND having it love you!

> *"Dress shabbily and they remember the dress.*
> *Dress impeccably and they remember you."*
>
> —Coco Chanel

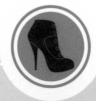

STEP UP TO ACTION:
No More Closet Chaos

1. Do I store both of my shoes together so I'm not wasting time trying to find the match?

2. What is my body shape?

3. What one thing do I need to implement as a closet chaos eliminator so that I can enjoy my morning routine more?

Chapter 10

SPARKLE AND SHINE, CREATING A LOOK THAT'S ALL MINE

"People are like stained-glass windows. They sparkle and shine when the sun is out, but when the darkness sets in, their true beauty is revealed only if there is a light from within."

—Elisabeth Kubler-Ross

Lace, leather, feathers, jewels, silk, cashmere, organic cotton, bobbles and bling, sophisticated, sporty, renegade, or cavalier? By now, you've surely discovered some hidden treasures in your closet and hopefully in your character that reflect your exclusive design. We've covered a lot of territory, and if you're still reading, then I truly hope you are ready to take yourself off the clearance rack of life and choose to value yourself for the one-of-a-kind woman that God—not the media or the woman on the treadmill next to you at the gym or even your mother—designed you to be.

Finding your unique way to sparkle and shine brings harmony to your life because it allows the contents of your container to shine through. Applying the principles in these chapters will help you go from naked to knockout daily with a style you've created, one that best expresses who you are and allows you to truly be comfortable in your own skin. Quit playing small by playing the comparison game, and quit giving up. You are worth so much more than you probably think.

If you are still struggling with looking in the mirror and *not* liking what you see, don't bust the mirror; bust the lie. Choose to see a knockout in that mirror if it means putting on boxing gloves and going to battle.

You'll be glad you took even one tiny baby step toward your image update. The rewards are really, really worth it. It will take you out of the 83% group who are unhappy with their body shape and catapult you to the 17% of happy campers.

Do I sound like a cheerleader? Maybe I do. . . . Maybe my seventh-grade practice sessions are still influencing my thoughts, but the point of cheering is to encourage progress and action, so let's talk about what's next.

A PONY OR A PILE?

The first step is to decide that there's a pony under a pile that you've accumulated (and we all have one). Perhaps it's a pile of negative self-talk or a pile of junk in the closet that needs to go, but I promise, if you're willing to dig for it, there's a pony waiting to step out in style.

Most women I work with hesitate when I get them too close to the edge of what they're used to, whether it's their lip color or style of skirt. Their protests usually sound like this: "But, Wendy, I couldn't dress like *that* or wear *that* color of lipstick because that whole 'sparkle and shine' thing just isn't me. And besides, I only work at or from home; no one even notices whether I dress up or not." Does that sound like you, too?

Well, honey, I've got a phrase for you: *we're fixin' to change that.* Every woman wants to sparkle and shine once she defines it for herself; unfortunately, too many women think that means being conservative to the point of boring (or invisible) or else standing out in a crowd like a pink elephant or a prancing peacock. As Stacy London, cohost of TLC's *What Not to Wear*, once remarked on the show, "It's as if you've never told the world who you are through the way you look." My point exactly.

SPARK TO ACTION

When you sparkle and shine, it's because the real you on the inside is aligned with the way you are presenting yourself on the outside, and yes, that probably means choosing to take at least one confident step out of your comfort zone. And then another . . . and maybe even another. It's a process, so, no, you don't have to do everything I've recommended by tomorrow afternoon . . . but doing at least one thing by then is a great way to start!

I hope you've taken advantage of the "Step up to Action" calls at the end of each chapter. If not, you might go back and look at how incorporating those suggestions will make a difference for you . . . or someone close to you. We are so full of impactful energy that making seemingly small changes in us and for "us" often has just as much impact (if not more) on those around us. So, it might even mean that the stay-home mom or work-from-home woman decides that it will benefit her bottom line with increased sales because her more confident voice on the phone will result in greater closings when she is dressed for success rather than in pj's or comfy sweats. It might also mean that motherhood has a dress code, too: dress as nicely as the women who work with your husband. As you giggle, I know you know it's true. You want him to like what he sees at home more than what he sees elsewhere!

Here are some more ideas.

1. Clear the piles; decide to clean out one category, such as your makeup and skin care products. Have they expired? Pitch them. Or clean out one section of your closet (slacks, shirts, etc.), looking for things that don't fit. What items cause you the most frustration? Choose to view it as an opportunity to make a change for the better.

2. Pal around: Share the concepts in this book with a friend so that together, you can do the face color test (holding up the white paper and the manila folder) and then edit your beauty products and clothing based on colors that work for you. Swap items that work better for the other person. Test the lipstick personality chart and have fun with glamour color. Listen for each other's negative self-talk and turn it into an opportunity to encourage each other. View the scarf-tying video and see whether you can share some accessorizing tips at your next "girls' night out" event. Receive a compliment with a simple

"thank you" rather than accounting for its bargain price. And, please, give compliments lavishly!

3. Identify the bargain boo-boos in your wardrobe. Turn them into opportunities for someone else to look her best by donating them to a women's shelter, for example. Create an S.O.S. bag to keep in your car: Save One's Sanity. Include items that are needed often but not on a daily basis (Band-Aids, tampons, stamps and postcards for good time management while you're "waiting," an extra pair of pantyhose, aspirin, spare earrings so you don't get caught "naked," clear nail polish, a house key, hairspray or a ponytail holder, a pen, and a $5 bill—I hate getting caught at tolls or needing that Starbucks). While the Internet has helped us become ever-so efficient, nothing replaces a handwritten note . . . It's a beautiful thing, so use that idle waiting time in the car line or at a doctor's office to bless someone with an old-fashioned, snail-mail note, written, of course, on some very stylish paper!

4. Write an encouraging note to a daughter, sister, friend, or mentor/ mentoree. Applying outwardly what you know inwardly builds self-confidence in a powerful way. And this is one small example of legacy building. Measure your contents-to-container ratio; does it need adjusting? If so, make it. Ask a trusted confidante for input and then together create some A-C-T . . . I-O-N. (Yes, that's another cheer!)

LOOK in the mirror and LIKE what you see . . . It gets easier when there's a positive connection between *what you're seeing* and *what you're saying.*

A TREASURE

In the Introduction, I listed three benefits you would receive from reading this book. Let's review.

No more needing to hide behind a mask of guilt, unworthiness, color un-know-how, and playing small to stay safe. Go out on a limb! That's where the fruit is, anyway. Most of our fears come with the idea of believing false evidence more than reality. It takes courage to push forward in the light of conflict. Conquering our fears pushes us out of our comfort zone behind the glass case and puts us on display. A treasure tends to be held in high esteem and "held" to a different light. Others view it with great awe. The value you attach to yourself is the one others will be drawn to. Respecting yourself as a treasure is the first step to having others treasure you too. Our Maker does that. The first benefit I hope you have received by reading this book is the ability to see yourself as a highly valuable and worthy of personal investments. Because of that, you will be able to embrace the relationships you have that are healthy and let others go. It's a simple philosophy of the law of attraction: a treasure attracts more of the same. Be a treasure. Share your distinctive gifts and talents with the world by expressing yourself exclusively.

The second benefit comes from knowing how to flatter your figure and organize your closet. When you do those two things better, your morning routine will be more peaceful, and who doesn't want that? You will save time and money when you buy what does work for you and stop buying what doesn't. Seeing a storyboard of tried-and-true, head-to-toe options will take a lot of the guesswork out of special-occasion dressing and make traveling light an easy task. Giving this area the attention it needs on the front end will save you time in the long run. Knowing where to shop saves you *even more time*. Window-shopping is fine for a stroll with a date, but power shopping results when price point and purpose align. Create some harmony and plan ahead so that you're not always stressing at the last minute about needed items.

Last, I trust that if you haven't already developed a style all your own, you can see one coming together. And don't change your style based on every new fad that comes out or at the request of every important person in your life. Be true to yourself, including putting your best face forward using the makeup tips, tricks, and tools mentioned here, whether you're going for a classic dash-out-the-door look or a dramatic and elegant one for glamour. Knowing how to reflect your personal style is easy when you know the message you want to convey.

Naked to Knockout: Beauty from the Inside Out is meant to help you save time getting dressed, create more healthy self-talk, provide smart makeup and hair how-to's, automatically accessorize any outfit to take it from good to great, and form better relationships. Implementing these, in turn, will help you slay the beast that may look back from the mirror and tempt you to wither away and pretend to be something you're not. When you do that, other people pick up on it more often than you might realize.

VICTIM OR VICTOR?

"I can absolutely get a feel from any woman I meet about her self-confidence level," says Kathleen Hawkins, author and founder of WOAMTEC, a national organization of networking for business women. Initial contact, body language, tonality, and smile—even if she has only a photo to look at—tell her whether a woman has inner strength. Amazingly, women can almost always sense when another woman is dressed to the nines with a shallow inside, as well as when a woman's personality and inner beauty are so strong that you hardly notice her average shell. Kathleen's experience comes from having worked with thousands of women who fit those two descriptions and from working with those who come out of the foster care system at age eighteen with practically nothing to offer the world except a background of neglect.

Women from all backgrounds and degrees of trauma still settle on common ground with their decision to be "victim" or "victor." Kathleen understands this; she was raised by a single parent, and choosing to survive, to be a victor, was really her only choice. She is a woman of faith who states openly that her definition of a beautiful woman would have to include someone living with a clear mission and purpose . . . a woman true to her virtues. When I asked what she does when faced with a challenge, she quickly answered, "That's easy. My mom always gave me three choices to make. **Fix it, live with it, or get rid of it.**"

That's a good bit of advice for adding some spark to your life. And speaking of spark, isn't it wild how the smallest efforts for good begin to attract more of the same? I have another friend whose life mantra is "Be a magnet for good." What she's basically saying is to assume an attitude of positive expectancy. Connecting your life mission and purpose with a cause has an incredible way of boosting your self-esteem. As the song goes, it only takes a spark to get a fire going. You never know how your freedom to excel, improve, and shine releases others to do the same.

LIGHTEN YOUR LOAD AND BURN, BABY BURN

Getting rid of some baggage along the way does a lot more than lighten your load . . . it adds fuel to the fire for an empowering spark to ignite. A spark is just the beginning of fire. We often hear about the horrific effects of fire spreading rapidly. Let's consider the positive benefits of fire: it warms, it causes others to be united as it draws a crowd, it's reflective, it requires oxygen to burn (breathe of life), it purifies elements and cooks food that provide nourishment for others. A human soul of fire cannot be easily quenched. The rage can spread rapidly to others providing more benefit *or detriment* . . . so be careful, everything intended for good has an evil side. It takes wisdom to know how to burn brightly for the right reason, at the right time to make a positive impact. Don't let your spark get out of control, but do throw off excess weight that may be smoldering your flicker and begin to shine brightly. It's what you were made do to.

CELEBRATE

Life is too short to get too caught up in looking through a magnifying glass and noticing every flaw, every brow hair that needs plucking, every extra pound, and each new increase in my smile lines. So while I am here, I choose to celebrate just the way I am. Room for improvement? Yes. Will I get better and better, every day in every way? Yes. But for today, let's celebrate life and celebrate others who share it with us. Don't count the day done until you've made the day count!

This journey will be over all too soon, and I want to have made worthwhile memories to treasure forever. Girlfriends who support, encourage, and inspire are valuable treasures to me. They come in various sizes, shapes, and colors, and their views and backgrounds add spice and freshness to my measly approaches to lots of things. I appreciate their courage to overcome incredible odds, to be heroes in their own way. This sisterhood of buoyancy has helped keep me floating on those days when the only place I was going was down a drain. That's when they plucked me out of that vortex and set me on dry ground. Sometimes a gentle hug was enough, and others times I've needed a firmer sittin' down and talkin' to. I really am grateful God didn't put me on an island to do this thing called life alone. Seeing others overcome obstacles only spurs me on to look for the opportunities that lie beyond whatever my challenge-du-jour might be. While my inner resolve may be strong, I am still swayed by peer pressure, and in this case, it's a good thing. Thank goodness I have girlfriends who pressure me into doing the right things; I hope you do, too. They challenge me to INjoy the moments, INspire others, be an INfluence, and get INNERgized daily. This quote by BJ Gallagher describes so many of you: "Valiant women of exceptional courage with enduring power to cope . . . taking each problem one day at a time and never giving up HOPE. You're brave-hearted women with great resilience and you lift each other so well . . . bonded by a common understanding each with a story to tell."

To my fellow sister entrepreneurs, mothers, consultants, and inspiring speakers, may your flair for people be greater than your flair for fashion. Serving them with excellence is what gives our work purpose. I believe we can do it with style and IN STYLE . . . a style all our own. Your influence to me is indeed an energizing force.

New Level? New Devil

If you still feel that your light is dim, who is it that's dimming it?

Naysayers and negative nellies are plentiful, and their voices can come from our own heads as well as from the mouths of friends. I urge you to mentally put up the hand that says, "Stop right there." Sometimes you will need to put it up physically, too. When you make a decision to kick it up a level, be ready. Joyce Meyer's saying is so true: "New level? New devil." The attacks that will most definitely come after you should be a welcome sign that at least you're moving in a worthy direction. Stand firm and continue making positive choices; it does pay off.

Some days our choices create better results than others, so be careful whom you're listening to. If you blow it today, let it go. Forgive. Tomorrow is another opportunity to make better decisions for success. Don't be too hard on yourself. Reach out and reach up for support and accountability. There's some simplicity and perspective provided when the Bible says, "Naked I came into this world, and naked I shall leave." What we do with the time between those two dashes matters! Furthermore, the in-between-the-dash time requires the wearing of some threads, so wear them well. See yourself as royalty. Head up, shoulders back, with pep in your step. Throw on some glitter and sequins and begin a new day regardless of the obstacles; you'll at least be shining, and *that* attitude, girlfriend, is one worth wearing daily.

Obstacle or opportunity? Choose opportunity, and let your N2K transformation begin!

Recommended Resources

Title/Category, Name, Web site

Etiquette Expert, Lynn Symonds, www.heritageacademyofeandp.com

Shoe Design, Barbara Thorton, www.designershoes.com

Fashionista for Plus Size, Susan L. Weber, www.grandstyle.com

Custom Closets, ORG by Design, www.orgbydesign.com

Eliminate Chaos Expert, Laura Leist, www.eliminatechaos.com

Professional Organizer, Lorie Marrero, www.clutterdiet.com

Deals and Steals, Fashion Blogger, www.thebudgetfashionista.com

Fashion Expert, Mary Lou Andre, www.dressingwell.com

Kids' Hair Help, Hairstyle Blogger, www.cutegirlshairstyles.com

Life Coach, Jenn Lee, www.coachjenlee.com

Undergarments, Spanx, www.spanx.com

Jewelry, A Lucky Find, www.aluckyfind.com

Hosiery, Silkies, www.silkies.com

Packing, Susan Foster, www.smartpacking.com

Travel Resource, Journey Woman, www.journeywoman.com

Clothing, Gear, Advice, Travelsmith, www.travelsmith.com

Women's Clothing and More, Stein Mart, www.steinmart.com

Women's Clothing, Ann Taylor, www.anntaylor.com

Designer Clothing, Chico's, www.chicos.com

Women's Clothing, Talbots, www.talbots.com

Designer Clothing, Cache, www.cache.com

Women's Career Dress Help, Dress for Success, www.dressforsuccess.org

Peak Talent and Modeling Agency, *with locations in Los Angeles, Las Vegas, Dallas, Miami, New York, and San Diego,* www.Peakmodels.com

Image, Modeling, Acting School of Winter Park, FL, www.lisamaile.com

Coaching: Wendy Lipton-Dibner, MA, President and Founder of Move People to Action and Bestselling Author of *Shatter Your Speed Limits: Fast-Track Your Success and Get What You Truly Want in Business and in Life, ,* www.ShatterYourSpeedLimits.com

Self-Defense Expert, David Nance, www.personalsafetyexpert.com

Healthy Diet, Suzanne Somers, www.sexyforever.com

American Gospel Singer, Mandisa, www.mandisaofficial.com

Singer and Speaker, Donna Leigh, www.donnaleighworship.com

Miscarriages and Preeclampsia, AmyRobbinsWilson, www.angelbabylullabies.com, www.mommyjingles.com

H.O.P.E., Help Other People Eat, www.hopetolive.com

National Women's Networking Group (WOAMTEC), www.woamtec.com

National Domestic Violence Hotline, www.thehotline.org

Women's Shelter of Central Florida (the Haven), www.havenlakesumter.org

BOOKS:

Mary Kay on People Management, Mary Kay Ash

Modeling Secrets Revealed, Natasha Duswalt
www.modelingsecretsrevealed.com

I Didn't Bargain for This, Mitzi Perdue

You've Got What It Takes, Marita Littauer

Thinking for a Change, John Maxwell

Bringing up Girls, Dr. James Dobson

Think, Lisa Bloom

Unlimited, Jillian Michaels

Sell Naked on the Phone, Joe and Dawn Pici

The Power of One, Debra Berg, www.nicenetwork.org

The Millionaire Messenger, Brenden Burchard

Little Black Book of Connections, Jeffrey Gittomer

ACKNOWLEDGMENTS

I am humbled by God's grace. It is ultimately his faithfulness to pursue me that has allowed anything good to come to pass. I am most grateful for my relationship with Jesus Christ and his love, for without that, I could never understand how to love others fully.

This book is dedicated to my family . . . but not just my immediate one. I consider many to be part of my extended family and will attempt to appreciate them. I am a blended product of so many who have been worthy examples to me. As a student and a teacher, I have many to thank.

Mom, Dad, Betty, Siggy, and Jeanne—thank you for understanding me and loving me and especially your support during this project. It would never be worth it to stand alone. You have taught me that family is an irreplaceable and valuable gift. I love each of you. Thank you for cheering me on to follow my dreams. To my late father-in-law, Terry, who taught me that beauty does come in many shapes and sizes and that we all have a right to create a "style all our own."

Mackenzie, may you always know that being God's girl makes you even more beautiful. Clothing yourself with godliness is the most beautiful way to get dressed every day. Daddy and I think there's no one more awesome than you!

Kendall, your zest for knowing what you want in life at such a young age will serve you well. May you come to know that a beautiful spirit is more important than beautiful shoes. In the meantime, thinking you are indeed Cinderella is fine with me. You rock our world, and we can't imagine it without you!

My sister, Nathalie, and Tommy and their family: your knockout style keeps me thinking out of the box and striving to improve. I love and respect you for being comfortable in your own skin no matter what company you're in.

To Bette Lord Hillman, your empowering belief in me the past twenty-five years has made all the difference. The style you exemplify as a wife, mother, and businesswoman is one I am proud to have adhered to. Thank you for your profound impact and friendship. Even though you walk the dog in stilettos, you taught me indeed that the "contents" are more important than the "container."

To my book coach and creative editor, Lee Owen, thank you for spurring me on, keeping me humble, guiding me to think, asking tough questions, and believing that this would actually come to fruition. I am so grateful to be the recipient of your extraordinary talent.

The support staff, proofreaders, and designers at Jenkins Group have been a joy to work with.

And to my personal assistant, Danielle: you have more than saved the day! Thank you for being just what I needed in the office to stay focused and looking good. Your serving me with excellence is a true gift.

To my dearest friends who have cheered me on: life is meant to be shared, and I can't imagine completing this project without your love, support, and prayers. I love you, Doria, Debra, MerryLee, Melanie, Kristin, Wendy P., Amy, Lee, Sharmin, and Gail.

To my consultants, customers, and sister directors, thank you for your loyalty, your feedback with questionnaires and e-mails, and your overall encouragement. You help me sweat pink glitter, and you have added much inspiration to my perspiration to see this to completion.

I so appreciate my church family, First Eustis, and their being an anchor for our family throughout life's trials and celebrations. The ultimate family of encouragement, you are!

To all my associates in business and all who have shared stories and data, given interviews, participated in focus groups, and worked your businesses with excellence, thank you for propelling me higher. I have learned from you that "if I have one good idea and you have one good idea and you share yours with me and vice versa, we both leave with two great ideas." Creating win-win relationships is really what it's all about. I love the collaborative process.

To the leaders in a plethora of industries who have truly paved the way for me to see a path of my own to travel, I admire and respect you. "Thanks" is a small word to say to giants such as Steve Harrison and the entire staff at Bradley Communications, too many Mary Kay Cosmetics directors and NSD's to mention, Wendy Lipton-Dibner, Rick Frishman, John Maxwell, David Cooper, Brendon Burchard, Ann McIndoo, and many other coaches.

Glenn, I love doing life with you . . . forever! You are a knockout in your own right, and it was that style that drew me to you. Thank you for being my best friend.